THE SMART SIMPLE GUIDE TO A BETTER PHYSIQUE

THE SMART SIMPLE GUIDE TO A
BETTER PHYSIQUE

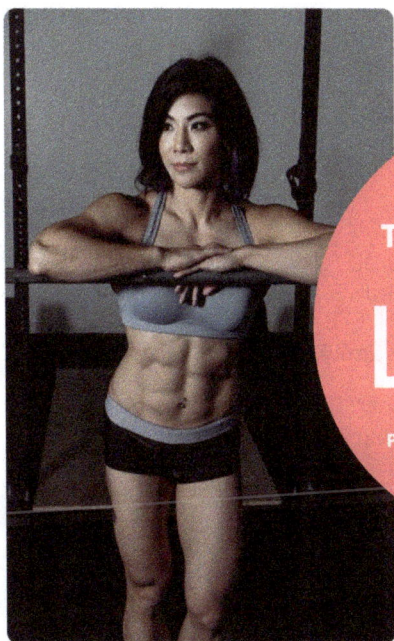

FITNESS, STRENGTH TRAINING, and NUTRITION **LESSONS** FROM A PROFESSIONAL ATHLETE AND BIOMEDICAL ENGINEER

EMILY HU, M.S.

THE SMART SIMPLE GUIDE TO A BETTER PHYSIQUE—
FITNESS, STRENGTH TRAINING, AND NUTRITION LESSONS
FROM A PROFESSIONAL ATHLETE AND BIOMEDICAL ENGINEER
By Emily Hu

Author and Publisher: Emily Hu, San Mateo, California, USA

ISBN e-Book: 979-8-218-12535-6
ISBN Paperback: 979-8-218-14331-2

ACKNOWLEDGMENTS

This book would not have been written without the encouragement of Emily Wang, who reminded me to keep writing as long as I found it fun, even if I was afraid that others might find the end result trite or corny.

Additionally, it would have been completely impossible for me to have written this book without the decade-long tutelage of Dan Green, who, the first time I wandered into a gym, said something to me along the lines of, "Whether you think you'll suck at it or not, you're going to have to learn how to bench press if you want to powerlift." Thanks to Dan, powerlifting victories and all-time world records suddenly entered into my realm of possibility, and it's been an amazing journey ever since.

Most importantly, a special thanks to my friends, family, and lifting crew who supported me every day, not only in writing this book, but in my lifting journey that ultimately led to its creation:

Eileen/Kaki, David, Shaun, Gracie, and the
Boss Barbell Crew

And some final thanks to Jordan Gruber, Marko Marković, Ryan Omega, Mike Dean, and Yi Yan for helping me bring this small book to the world.

LEGAL, MEDICAL, AND SAFETY DISCLAIMER

The author and publisher has no medical training or formal credentials in any medical or fitness area, practice, or specialty. While this book provides carefully researched and thoughtfully considered information, based on both published studies and personal experience, it is impossible for it to address the unique health history and medical condition of each and every individual reader.

Therefore, before starting any new or revised exercise program or making any substantial dietary changes, please discuss your plans with your personal health care provider.

Please understand that the author cannot be held responsible for individual accidents or injuries that might come about from any individual reader's actions or adaption of this book's information to their own individual circumstances. Nor can the author be responsible for any accidents, injuries, or mishaps that happen from the unintended, unconscious, or unsafe use of any exercise equipment or dietary protocol.

It's your job to keep yourself—and those who come in contact with you—safe.

So good luck, stay safe, and have fun as you become healthier, stronger, and happier on your personal journey towards a better physique and greater fitness.

TABLE OF CONTENTS

INTRODUCTION

All right, you picked up this book! Some of you may have been down this road before. You may have tried different diets, workouts, and possibly even a miracle pill or three. Perhaps you've read or listened to some books—or at least the latest online articles and podcasts—and you're just not getting the results you want. Or maybe—including those of you who are beginners—you just want clear, easy directions that take the guesswork out of the process of getting fit and healthy and can guarantee some real results.

And it's not just you. Over the course of the COVID pandemic, several of my friends who had become sedentary and gained weight during San Francisco's prolonged shelter-in-place mandate reached out to ask me, "How can I get into shape quickly?" After giving the same basic advice to ten friends, I started writing down my thoughts and sharing the document. The more I shared, the more follow-up questions I ended up answering, until what started as an online document began to resemble a book. This book, in fact. I hope it might help you as much as it did them.

My first response to "How can I get into shape quickly?" was *not* a list of difficult things to do that demonstrate how hard it is to get fit. Instead, I always tell people that achieving a basic level of fitness can be pretty easily worked into a busy schedule if you are willing to make a few lifestyle changes and be wise about your time. (In my own case, people are often surprised that I work in the biotech industry with a 40+ hour work week, which includes regular travel, whereupon I'm occasionally a glutton for food...but not for punishment.)

This book does not promote some puffed-up version of "fitness is a lifestyle" and "you need to give 110%" to achieve results. Unless you are a professional athlete—in which case you wouldn't need this book—then fitness is, at best, a part of your life, and not your whole life.

One principle that we will come back to time and again is this one:

Work Smarter, Not Harder

Regularly doing 100 sit-ups thinking you will get you a six-pack may seem logical, but thanks to science, we know it's just not the case (otherwise, you would have done that and this would have been a very short book). So let's give you a set of tools that actually works—and the knowledge needed to use them—so your efforts produce real progress!

Better Late Than Never

Like many of you, I did not get serious about my fitness journey until later in life. I was 30 years old the first time I powerlifted. I know our circumstances will be somewhat different: in my case, I transitioned from being a relatively fit person to a first-time competitive athlete at what is considered a geriatric age for an athlete. In your case, you may be an adult who's hoping to level up from couch potato to gym enthusiast, or maybe you're already pretty fit but want to take your physique to the next level.

Whatever your starting point, trust me when I tell you that I know starting the journey can feel overwhelming, especially when you have no idea how the journey is supposed to look. Mine started off with fairly modest goals: I only wanted to learn how to properly deadlift because I thought competing in my first athletic competition would be a fun new thing to try at the age of 30. Even then, I found every excuse in the world to wait 6 months before signing up for my first powerlifting competition. Every competition was either "on an inconvenient weekend" or "too close to me returning from a vacation," but the truth is I was really just too nervous to even start. I eventually hired a wiser and more experienced person to help me get through the process, and not only did I win on the day of my first powerlifting meet, but I broke every state record in my weight class!

While your fitness journey may not lead you to competing, I still hope my story can serve as an example: small beginnings can lead to surprising results, even if fitness isn't your sole focus. I'd like to believe that my story also demonstrates that new endeavors—such as my success as an athlete—are made easier with help, be it coaching or additional resources.

WHY AM I WORTH LISTENING TO?

- I'm a three-time world record holder in powerlifting, a national level Olympic weightlifter and bodybuilder who had a full-time tech career the entire time. I went from picking up weights—not completely sure what I was doing—to becoming an all-time world record holder with professional sponsorships in 3 years, to being recruited by NBC for Dwayne "The Rock" Johnson's *The Titan Games.*

- I have a master's degree in Biomechanical Engineering from Duke University. A good portion of my career has been spent as a researcher conducting human subject research in orthopedics (in which I published a scientific paper on knee pain) and physical medicine, so, naturally, my coursework and work experience have given me a detailed understanding of human biomechanics.

- Early in my powerlifting career, I earned a nutrition certification from Cornell University so I could serve as my own nutritionist. I started off trying out a few different nutrition coaches but found their programs too rigid for someone with a really busy life outside of lifting. Basically, I took evening courses so I could manage my own nutrition.

- In my 10 years as a competitive athlete, I've trained under coaches with different specialties, many of whom were experts in their field.

- And—most importantly—I achieved all of this while not being a career athlete or fitness industry worker, just like the vast majority of adults trying to improve their strength and physiques.

I'm confident that my background and experience demonstrate that I have some insight to share. But like most people, my daily life has consisted of challenges that sometimes made my fitness journey daunting or intimidating:

- As a child and teenager, I didn't receive the kind of proper athletic training I could take into adulthood. I didn't compete in sports in high school or college, and my first powerlifting competition was also the first time I had attended any sort of weightlifting competition. Prior to that, I'd never seriously trained for anything. So when I say that I went in blind, let me tell you, I really had no idea about what was involved with powerlifting or athletic training.

- The entire time I was training as a professional powerlifter, including my time preparing for and filming NBC's *The Titan Games*, I did it alongside a full-time job in biotech. My career has always been my first priority, with my lifting life second. So please know that even if you can't make fitness your highest priority, you can still do a really good job without a superhuman effort.

- I traveled for work constantly (up to 3 weeks a month and up to three cities a week), so meal prepping, and eating or lifting at specific times each day, was usually not possible. During work trips with colleagues or clients, you don't get to control what time you eat, let alone where you eat most times. I had to learn the most efficient ways to be flexible given my unpredictable work life. Admittedly, I also don't handle stress very well, so after a very long day of traveling to random cities and hospitals to conduct medical tests, the last thing I'd want to do was force myself to eat tilapia and broccoli!

- This is definitely not any sort of brag, but rather an admission, that I have a weakness in sticking to routines and plans. My coaches will tell you that I'm both a hardworking *and* noncompliant athlete; I'll work really hard on the things that I find necessary or interesting, but then I'll cut a lot of corners elsewhere. Maybe it's my ADHD, but I hate routines and diets which are overly restrictive or too involved. I need flexibility to not feel overwhelmed or bored. For this reason, I've designed a good deal of flexibility into the programs and routines I recommend.

10 YEARS OF COACHING— THE BIGGEST HITS...REMIXED!

In many strength sports, including the three I've competed in, it's fairly common to hire a coach for your nutrition as well as a coach for your actual workout. Often these are two different people. Even with my occasional extreme noncompliance, I was able to learn a lot from each of my coaches and, over time, combine their best lessons into practical execution.

That's what I'm offering you here, my distilled knowledge and experience from 10 years of coaches and coaching, the best and biggest hits. But first, there are some disclaimers associated with this approach that we need to briefly discuss before getting into the rest of the book.

For starters, if you want a book on the current state of exercise or nutrition science, there are more qualified resources you should turn to. This book is not a science or fitness book. This is not a diet book. This is more of a synthesized diary of tips and shortcuts that seem to work pretty well on myself and most healthy people than it is a presentation of scientific or nutritional theories or systems.

While the outcomes that have informed my decisions and ultimately this book are based on science, the solutions that I present are merely simplifications made through applying my scientific background to my experiences and observations. None of the advice I'm going to give you here is new or novel, but for you personally, it might represent a discovery and make an important difference.

This book also assumes that you are a normal and physically healthy individual with no underlying medical conditions. If that's not the case, ask a healthcare professional how you can incorporate elements of this guide into your own lifestyle.

Now, you might ask, "Isn't fitness mainly predetermined by genetics? You know, some of us have it and some of us don't. And obviously, you have it..." Indeed, many people think that they can't achieve fitness because they simply don't have the genetics (or the metabolism, which we'll come to in a minute).

In my case, it is true that:

- My father was a collegiate rugby player. I have his same broad stature so maybe I'm naturally stronger than most women.

- I had disposable income the whole time I was training so I could afford to hire the best help.

- I've never been severely out of shape or overweight. Even during my heavier and fitness naive years, I still had a gym membership where I regularly (and inefficiently) lifted tiny brightly colored dumbbells and used the elliptical machine.

But keep in mind that:

- I was 30 when I started. Prior to this, I had never competed in sports.

- I had a busy full-time job the whole time; I missed multiple days—sometimes weeks—of training due to work travel and long workdays.

- I have an incredibly average metabolism. If I don't work out or watch what I eat, I put on weight easily. I've even undergone metabolic testing at a medical clinic that determined that my resting metabolism was completely average for my height, weight, and age.

- I have ADHD. Some people think this is an advantage. In some ways, it is: if I really love something, like powerlifting, I can work *very* hard at it (during these moments, everyone will tell you that I have a great work ethic). In every other way, it is an absolute weakness; my ADHD is easily my own worst enemy. I can't stick to a diet or a routine, I'll cut corners if I find them boring, and I'm terrible at following directions. Most sport training requires some amount of repetitiveness and I HATE it. There were many times in my own training that I went rogue, to my own detriment, just because I was so bored to death with the routine.

The point here: I was pretty average—maybe even below average—up until the day I wasn't. Sure, I worked out regularly and was pretty healthy even before powerlifting, but before age 30, no one would have ever looked at me and thought, "Yeah, that lady is a world-class athlete."

Anyone can be fitter, leaner, stronger, and healthier than they were yesterday. Anyone can develop a better physique. Sometimes, you can become a lot more than you ever thought possible. And yes, I mean even you.

Also, keep in mind that no one here is expecting you to become a champion powerlifter because you read this book; I'm just hoping to make diet and exercise a little less mysterious and a lot more doable.

HOW THIS BOOK IS LAID OUT

First, we'll look at Food, then Exercise and Movement, then Sleep, and finally Supplements.

FOOD—There are a lot of opinions on what foods to eat or not eat. While the Internet is a great source for finding ample information, it's not so good at helping you discern what's true from what's a food fad. Keep in mind that search engines generally support our own confirmation biases (search for information on any food plan and you'll find some site that supports it without citing any evidence). We also have those friends who claim they've lost 15 lbs. cutting carbs, or meat, or "foods that start with S," and have a special plan that worked for them. But did they keep the weight off? So here, we'll discuss what worked for me while dropping some validated scientific knowledge along the way.

EXERCISE AND MOVEMENT—This section is called "Exercise and Movement" because when some people see the word "Exercise" in this kind of book, they put up mental roadblocks like "this is too hard" or "this is not for me" before even starting. The reality is that any movement is better than none, and most of us already undertake some movement, including whenever we walk to the office or the grocery store. With that said, before we buy the latest fitness contraption that more resembles fetish gear than home gym equipment, remember that *most effective exercises are simple and have become long-time staples because they actually work well.* And if you get bored easily or get very busy, like I sometimes do, you'll have multiple options as to when you can perform the activities you pick.

> *"Most effective exercises are quite simple and have become long-time staples only because they actually work well."*

SLEEP—If you're looking for the most effective and efficient way to become fit, this is your key right here! If you haven't had much progress in getting fit or losing weight, look at how much sleep you are getting. Your mind might have every intention to work out and eat right, but if you don't have enough sleep, your body won't cooperate and can sabotage your best-laid plans. So ultimately, if your body is the thing you want to change, you may have to treat it like a cranky two-year-old child who has demands... and needs, like more sleep.

SUPPLEMENTS—Looking for magic pills? Many of us have tried versions of diet stimulants, laxatives, or even capsules derived from some exotic Asian herb that promises more energy and weight loss. There are definitely some supplements that will enhance your progress; I'll tell you which ones and describe how they work (not according to magic, but according to science).

As for what's *not* here, if you were expecting a big chapter on motivation or discipline, no doubt you're already well aware of your own reasons, and those will be far more powerfully motivating than anything I can spell out in writing. Whether it's looking good at the beach or family reunion, wanting to fit into your favorite outfit again, or desiring more energy throughout the day, please keep your reasons strong in your mind as you mine the information you need from this guide and put it to use.

In summary, if you're looking for a way to create a fitter body and better physique, then these main sections—Food, Exercise & Movement, Sleep, and Supplements—will serve as your primary set of personal keys to the kingdom. So let's go ahead and dive into food.

PART 1

FOOD

Over and over, I've found that what's most helpful is to empower someone with the information and knowledge they need to make their own best decisions.

I'm well aware that by now, some of you may be looking for "eat" and "don't eat" lists that you can stick on your fridge... and then be done. These lists may be all that you want, but if you look at your life, how easy is it to follow such lists when you're hanging out with friends who want to go to the new downtown Italian restaurant, or when you find yourself at a big family holiday meal?

Moreover, many of us don't like being told what to do, myself included. We have an internal block that goes something like, "If it's too restrictive at all, it becomes a chore, and I just don't have the mental energy for that."

Instead of dictating what someone should do when it comes to food, I find that it is far more helpful to empower someone with the information and knowledge they need to make their own best decisions. That is, I will tell you how your body works, explain why many diet plans have failed, and then show you how to make smarter choices, all without always having to return to a bookmarked section in this guide or some other resource.

If you read through, understand, and apply this information—maybe not all of the time, but at least some of the time—then you'll find yourself making far more progress. Before we turn to the main course and dive into macronutrients (and fiber!), let's look at two common assumptions or sayings that many people have in their head, and see whether they contain a kernel of truth or perhaps need some additional context.

TWO COMMON ASSUMPTIONS

Assumption # 1: "Abs are made in the kitchen"

Luckily for you, you can get a pretty nice physique working out three to four times per week. This is because the biggest contributor to your physique is your diet. The silver lining here is that during times when you are too busy to get in a workout, you can still make big strides in improving your body composition if you are able to maintain a somewhat healthy diet.

Unfortunately for the "I want to get a six pack" crowd, this also means that you can't just do sit-ups to get flat, chiseled abs. Ultimately, losing weight is how abdominal muscles become most visible. This is more affected by *what you eat* than by *how much strain you put on your muscles*, which is why a significant portion of this book is about food.

Here's the thing: while no one can force you to work out, as a human being, you *have to* eat to stay alive. I'll show you how the quality of your food is just as important as the quantity of those calories.

Assumption # 2: "You can't outrun a bad diet"

A lot of people believe that if you exercise enough, you can eat whatever you like, and as much as you like. While I wish this were true, practically speaking, it just isn't. Unless you're an ultra-marathoner, given how heavily caloric so many foods in the Western diet are, there's very little chance you can exercise enough to counterbalance truly poor food choices.

Sadly, exercise doesn't burn as many calories as we tend to think it does. Not only that, we tend to eat a lot more calories than we think we do.

For example, a 125 lb. woman burns about 100 calories jogging 1 mile. A 200 lb. man burns about 200 calories during the same activity. This means that for one hour of nonstop jogging, the same woman burns about 500 calories, and the man burns about 1,000. Consider that one large slice of Domino's pepperoni pizza is approximately 300 calories (and let's be real, no one eats just one slice), a medium order of fries from McDonald's is 400 calories, mozzarella sticks are about 100 calories each, and a margarita at a restaurant is about 300 calories.

Let's say you go to happy hour with friends and have just two drinks, three mozzarella sticks, and two slices of pizza. That's a meal in the ballpark of 1,500 calories—that's almost an entire day's worth of calories for a 125 lb. woman! You haven't even had your "I'm tipsy, let's grab some McDonald's on the way home" fries yet! That's about an hour and a half run for the man to balance this out, and a three-hour run for the woman. But can you run like that every time you go out to eat? Probably not. The better question is, why would you even want to? Instead, we want to focus on keeping down the total number of calories being consumed in the first place.

Yes, we're also going to address how being taller, older, or even biologically female or male makes some of this easier or less easy (fairer or unfairer) for different people, because everyone's biology is different. A "one-size-fits-all" strategy fits only one person, so we'll be looking at different ways to find out what works best for you. Now let's turn to Macronutrients (and Fiber!).

MACRONUTRIENTS (AND FIBER!)

It's important to start with a good look at the science of food. We've been conditioned to think that fat is bad, and that sometimes carbs are bad too. But before we label any part of any food as "good" or "bad," let's look at how those parts actually *function*, and then leverage those functions to serve our goals!

One important piece of diet vocabulary as we get started is the idea of "macronutrients"—or "macros" for short—which are the nutritive components our bodies require in large amounts. For human beings, there are three types of macros: fats, proteins, and carbohydrates.

Fat

Fat is the most calorically dense macronutrient. It contains more than twice the calories per gram when compared to carbs or protein, so cutting fat first goes a long way. However, while in one sense fat may be "the enemy," it also serves important functions in our bodies.

Fats are needed to regulate hormones such as estrogen, testosterone, and thyroid hormones. Too little fat and our endocrine system—responsible for our hormones—can't function optimally, potentially leading to irritability, fatigue, and even low libido! Hormonal imbalance not only affects your mood and metabolism but can make you susceptible to diseases and otherwise interfere with your well-being.

Another reason for not fully cutting out fat completely is that it also contributes to optimal brain function. Not only is your brain nearly 60 percent fat by weight, but fatty acids are what's used to help maintain the structure and functions of the brain's different types of cells.

One more important reason your diet should contain fat is that it is more difficult for the stomach to absorb, so calories from fat are digested more slowly than calories from other macronutrients. A little fat with every meal will help keep you feeling satiated and full!

You might have heard that there are "good" fats and "bad" fats, otherwise known as unsaturated (the good), saturated (the bad), and trans (the ugly) fats. We'll go into detail later about how to use good fats to your advantage, but first, let's explain what makes fat "good" or "bad."

Monounsaturated and polyunsaturated fats, also known as **unsaturated fats,** are what we tend to call "good fats." Research has shown that eating foods that contain good fats can help protect your heart by maintaining blood levels of "good" HDL cholesterol while reducing levels of "bad" LDL cholesterol. Foods high in good fats include avocado, nuts, seeds, and fish.

Eating too much "bad fat"—such as **saturated fats**—can raise the LDL cholesterol in your blood, which can increase the risk of heart disease and stroke. Foods high in saturated fats include red meat, full-fat dairy products, and coconut.

Even more harmful than saturated fats are **trans fats**. Trans fats increase the risk of heart attacks, stroke, and type 2 diabetes, even when eaten in small quantities. Trans fats are primarily found in deep fried foods and processed foods made with partially hydrogenated oil such as refrigerated dough, packaged cookies, margarine, and coffee creamer.

Protein

This macronutrient is most commonly associated with meat and serves as the building block of all cellular growth and repair in our body. After a hard workout, it's the amino acids in the protein that we eat that repair and grow the muscle. The body also uses protein to maintain most of its functions (think muscle, bone, hair, nail, skin, etc.) and systems including digestion, hormone production, blood clotting, and immune system function.

Protein is actually the best macronutrient to help you feel full despite what fans of the Keto Diet believe. While fat may be more difficult to digest, eating protein reduces your body's level of the hormone ghrelin, the hormone which makes you feel hungry, thus decreasing your hunger. While fat stops you from eating more when you are eating, protein ensures that you don't have intense hunger signals in the first place!

However, not all protein is created equal: eggs, beef, and dairy products have the highest bioavailability (which means how much your body can absorb and use) for muscle repair and growth, while plant proteins like beans and peas have less bioavailability (typically 25%–75%) because not only is up to 20% of the plant protein indigestible, but the amino acid profile of the proteins in these plants does not quite match the needs of the human body. For those looking to build muscle, plant proteins are less effective. To give you an example of indigestibility, sometimes after we eat food and excrete, when what comes out looks similar to the food we ate, it is because the body was not able to entirely break down the food. (If you have eaten corn, you likely know this experience....)

Carbohydrates

Carbohydrates ("carbs") are a macronutrient that function mostly as an energy source and are synonymous with starch or sugar. Carbohydrates are commonly found in breads, pasta, rice, and fruit, but also in vegetables. To oversimplify, the carbs we eat are broken down into sugars, which then enter our bloodstream to provide our body with its quickest source of energy. (The next quickest energy source is protein, then fat.)

Carbs get a bad rap because when their broken-down sugars enter our blood stream, it causes a rise in the infamous "blood sugar levels" that we so often hear about. Eating large amounts of carbs leads to a surge in blood sugar, which the body quickly works to lower. This results in blood sugar dropping rapidly, which feels like a sudden drop in energy or a "sugar crash." Frequent blood sugar surges like these are known to increase your chances of diabetes. However, carbs are not inherently bad for you as long as you maintain some semblance of balance in your diet; we'll look at this again a little later on.

Carbs are also very important for athletic performance and muscle growth: you can't work hard if you don't have any energy! The more strenuous the activity, the more your body will rely on carbs for energy, so unless you mainly plan on lying around on your couch all day, I'd suggest that you keep some amount of carbs in most meals (more on this later).

You need protein and fat to stay alive and keep your body functioning. It is possible but not fun to survive without carbs. Put differently, if you are just trying to lose weight, carbs are the least important macronutrient group, so if you don't care about athletic performance, you can cut them the most.

If you are working out regularly, you can reduce carbs without cutting them out completely, but this will greatly diminish your energy level thereby also reducing the quality of your workouts. So definitely do not remove carbs from your pre-workout meal, or your workouts (and you!) will really suffer. You'll also want to keep some carbs in your post workout meal to replenish your energy levels.

"Speaking of carbs, aren't natural sugars supposed to be healthier than white sugar?"

Many food companies and fad diets state that natural sugars such as honey, agave syrup, and maple syrup are healthier for you than white sugar because they are "natural," but this is really just a marketing gimmick. Yes, natural sugars may contain some nutrients that processed white or brown sugars do not, and some may cause slightly less of a blood sugar spike than others, but all of these products, including processed sugars, are constituted of a mix of glucose and fructose. In short, "sugar is sugar is sugar." Once you normalize the serving size, all sugar products contain the same amount of calories and carbs per serving.

For example, honey is sweeter than white sugar but it also has more calories per teaspoon. While you would need less honey to make your cup of tea as sweet, you would still be consuming the same number of carbs and calories as if you had added sugar. This is not meant to dissuade you from using natural sugars if you enjoy them—by all means, enjoy! Just know that when it comes to dieting, this book will treat every type of sugar the same, whether it is natural or processed.

Fiber

Fiber is most commonly associated with fruits and vegetables. While fiber is technically not a macronutrient, it's just as important a part of your diet, not only because it helps us go to the bathroom but because it's wonderful for health and longevity in general. An analysis of hundreds of scientific research studies has shown that a daily intake of 25–29 grams of dietary fiber is associated with lower weight, blood pressure, blood sugar, cholesterol, and lower risks of developing (and dying from) diabetes, heart disease, strokes, and breast or colon cancer. The American Heart Association recommends eating 25 to 30 grams per day of fiber with one-fourth—6 to 8 grams per day—coming from soluble fiber. It is fine to exceed this amount, but I would recommend that you spread your fiber intake across meals, even if you aren't eating more than the recommended amount, to reduce any resulting flatulence or bloating.

There are two types of fiber. First, **soluble fiber** is found in many fruits and vegetables. It is good for you for many reasons:

- It lowers the body's fat absorption, helping you to lose weight.

- It lowers cholesterol by preventing some dietary cholesterol from being absorbed into your bloodstream, potentially lowering your LDL (bad) cholesterol and improving cardiovascular health.

- It stabilizes blood sugar (glucose) levels by slowing down the digestion rate of carbohydrates, thereby reducing or preventing spikes in blood sugar

Next, **insoluble fiber** is found in some vegetables (like cauliflower and dark leafy greens), beans, and grains. Its primary benefit is that it increases bowel health, but it also helps you feel fuller longer just by taking up physical space in your stomach, helping you to consume less of other, more highly caloric foods.

WHY FAD DIETS WORK
(BUT ONLY FOR A WHILE)

Before turning to how I successfully lose weight, let's look at some of the most popular fad diets and see why they fail in the long run.

How many fad diets have you tried? For me, it's been quite a few. Back in college, I tried a few 2-day "liquid cleanses" in hope of "dropping 5–10 pounds overnight!" No one tells you that the only weight you are losing is temporary water weight that returns the second you eat again. As an adult, I found that I could successfully lose some weight with intermittent fasting as long as I didn't need to work out that same day. If I did work out, however, I was often either too hungry or too bloated (depending on how close I was to my fasting window) to have a consistent workout.

At the end of the day, all diets work the same way—by putting you in a calorie deficit. Fad diets, to the degree that they work at all, do so because they are based on making entire types or kinds of food unavailable. That is, eliminating a food group means there is less that you can eat overall, so it becomes relatively easy to move into a calorie deficit. But again, there is nothing inherently fat burning about eating only fat or drinking only juice.

Moreover, the side effects from eliminating entire food groups can be really harsh. Even though you might lose weight temporarily, no one talks about the malnutrition or muscle loss from keto or veganism, developing insulin resistance from high carb meals, compromising your heart health from high fat diets, or long-term sustainability and overall health impacts generally.

Let's now review some current fad diets and their limitations.

Cutting Out Meat: Vegan/Vegetarian Diet

Removing animal products means there is less protein in your diet. I understand when people choose a vegan/vegetarian diet for sustainability and moral reasons, but if you are doing it because you think it is healthier, then it's time to pick up your steak knife again.

Vegetarianism as a method for weight loss assumes that all meat is inherently more fatty than non-meat foods. Veganism similarly assumes all animal products are more fatty than plant-based foods. Neither assumption is necessarily true: chicken breast, turkey breast, and shellfish are much leaner and thus have less calories per serving than the more common vegetarian or vegan protein substitutions in prepared foods, which are full-fat dairy products or seeds and nuts, respectively. Additionally, some plant-based food alternatives actually have more fat and calories per serving than the original version. A number of plant-based ground beef alternatives contain just as many calories per serving while having more fat and saturated fat than lean ground beef. Cashew cheese contains about 20 more calories per ounce than regular goat cheese, plus nearly double the amount of total fat.

Another challenge with these diets is that the bioavailability of non-animal protein is somewhat low (in general, 75% or less unless the protein is processed) so you won't build a lot of muscle if you're concerned about athletic performance or your physique. Also, since you have fewer options for protein, you're more likely to eat more fat to feel full—and fat, remember, is higher in calories. Think about it, what are the vegetarian options at your local restaurant? A cheese pizza? Fettuccine Alfredo? Both of those are far more caloric and less nutrient dense than grilled chicken or fish. For all of these reasons, many people who become vegetarians or vegan might lose weight during the first few weeks of the diet, but actually end up gaining weight after those first few weeks.

"I'm a vegan; can I still get buff?"

Of course you can! But you will need to put in a little extra planning and effort to get adequate protein with every meal. My suggestion would be to avoid nuts as your main protein source as they are very fatty with low protein bioavailability (most nuts contain at least twice as much fat as they do protein) and instead choose legume proteins with the highest bioavailability, such as soybeans (tofu or tempeh) and chickpeas. However, keep in mind that unlike with meat, legume-based plant proteins contain a lot of carbs, so you will need to factor that into your meal's total macronutrient count: one serving of 25 g of soy protein will contain half a serving of carbs, while for chickpeas it's two servings. So your entire meal might end up being just tofu with veggies, or chickpeas and salad with some avocado.

Another thing to keep in mind is that both of these plant proteins still have somewhere around 75% protein bioavailability so you may need to eat a little more than one serving to truly absorb 25 g of protein. So, if building muscle without gaining too much fat is a priority, it would be beneficial to supplement some of your meals with plant-based protein powders to boost your protein intake. Otherwise, you may find yourself eating more calories in carbs than you intended just to hit your protein goal. When going the protein powder route, I recommend soy protein powders as well as rice and pea protein blends as their processing leaves the protein more digestible with bioavailability increased to almost 90%.

Cutting out Carbs: The Keto (Ketogenic) Diet

A true Keto Diet means that 75% or more of your calories must come from fat and less than 5% from carbs. Carbs per meal must be very low to not raise your blood sugar; that means limiting your intake of grains, starchy veggies, beans, lentils, fruits, vegetables, and dairy products. Doing this results in nutrient and fiber deficiencies. Moreover, when a diet is high in saturated fat, it can increase your risk of heart disease, especially if you don't exercise. If you do exercise, there is not enough protein allowed in this diet for muscle building. Also, no carbs means no quick energy for your muscles during an intense workout, so your speed and strength will be reduced, and your regular workout will feel a lot harder relative to when you are carbed up.

The Atkins Diet

This is a similar high-fat/low-carb diet that lets you have more protein than the Keto Diet along with a reduction of fat. Nonetheless, with Atkins the potential heart disease risks and negative impacts on your workouts are similar to the keto diet.

One of the major underlying beliefs for followers of either of these diets is that not just sugar, but all carbs, make you fat. The truth is, any macronutrient can make you fat if consumed in excess, not just carbs; there is no macronutrient group that is inherently more fattening than the others when you control for calories.

Cutting Out All Solid Foods: Juice Fasts Or Any Liquid Cleanse

It's wonderful to eat fruits and vegetables with other food because they are both low calorie and full of fiber, which helps keep you full and prevents you from eating more caloric food. Despite the claims of juicing advocates, when you are just drinking the juice of something, you simply don't get the full benefit. Moreover, with juice fasts—in which you replace entire meals with fruit or vegetable juices—you get instant carbs to the bloodstream that can cause a subsequent sugar crash. Drinking juice on an empty stomach quickly raises your blood sugar. This is something that those concerned about diabetes might want to avoid.

Also, the act of digestion not only sends signals of satiety to your brain, but also plays a sizable role in your metabolism. So if you are only drinking liquids, your metabolism will slow down. This, combined with no fiber, protein, or fat, will leave you feeling very hungry all the time.

Also, on juice fasts and liquid cleanses, your daily fat and protein intake typically drop to zero. For reasons we've already covered, this is not great for your hormones, muscles, or bones.

Cutting Out All Foods: Intermittent Fasting

This diet only works because it serves as a means to reduce the number of hours you can eat and does not increase your metabolism in any way. Eating only one very large meal a day is not great for maintaining energy levels, and it is not optimal for digestion. Individual meals under intermittent fasting plans are likely to be larger than non-fasting meals, and if you are eating two of those meals in one day, the first meal may be too large to be fully digested before the next meal. Not only that, but since you're ravenously hungry going into your eating window, you are more likely to consume more food than you might during a normal eating day. It should also go without saying that the absence of food will have a negative impact on your workouts: many studies have shown that athletes perform significantly worse when they train during a fasting period. These factors combined make this diet tough for exercise enthusiasts: to have a good workout, you need to precisely time your workouts relative to your eating window so that you are neither too hungry nor too full.

Cutting Out All Foods Post-Stone Age: The Paleo Diet[1]

The Paleolithic (or "Paleo") Diet does not allow refined sugar, salt, legumes, dairy products, or processed foods and consists only of meat, fish, and plants. The diet stems from the idea that this is what ancient people ate. It boldly assumes that Paleolithic people were healthier than we are because our bodies have trouble digesting processed food.

However, realistically speaking, cavemen were *not* healthier than us nor did they live longer—they generally only lived between 25 and 35 years, and they didn't get certain diseases mainly because they died before the age that these diseases typically emerge. And, of course, generally they were hyper-lean—because they were malnourished and starving. Let's be real, hunting ungulates and gathering non-poisonous fruit is harder than hunting the local Costco for packaged meat and gathering a packaged box of Hass avocados.

Plants and animals, just like humans, have evolved and changed over time. It's pretty safe to say that the animals, fruits, and vegetables that the Paleolithic people ate are nothing like today's equivalents. (For reference: look up what a watermelon looked like in the 17th century compared to what we see today!) Paleo only works because it's very restrictive, not because it's healthier than any other diet. Aside from this diet being entirely based on marketing gimmicks instead of rational thought, this diet can be problematic for

---

[1]   See how ridiculous these elimination strategies are getting?

athletes, as the only source of pre-workout carbs allowed are from potatoes and fruit, which can be quite limiting.

The Raw Diet: Cutting Out Everything Processed, Eating Food Only In Its Original Form

The raw diet involves eating only unprocessed, uncooked plants such as fruits, vegetables, nuts, and seeds. The rationale is that cooking food destroys its nutrients. While this is partially true, cooking food does not destroy *all* its nutrients. Food can be cooked and still be quite healthy. We can also always cook food for shorter durations or at lower temperatures (such as steaming and sautéing instead of deep frying) so that minimal nutrients are destroyed by the heat.

This diet mostly works because it's so restrictive. As the *most* restrictive of all the diets we will look at, it is wildly impractical for most people. While eating more raw fruits and vegetables is always good for you, following this diet may leave you malnourished in terms of protein, calcium, iron, other vitamins and nutrients, and healthy fats. The typical raw vegan diet is so low in protein that you may actually lose both bone and muscle mass if you remain on it too long.

The Whole 30 Diet

The Whole 30 Diet may be healthy for some people, in some circumstances, but it's also pretty close to an unhealthy extreme elimination diet. The Whole 30 starts by eliminating several major types of foods, and then slowly reintroduces them into your diet. The selling premise is that since it only lasts 30 days, you can just "do a diet for a month." The Whole 30 cuts out all processed foods as well as grains, dairy, legumes, soy, and any added sugars or sweeteners, leaving you with meat, fruit, vegetables, and nuts. Because the diet is so restrictive, you will indeed lose weight. Much like with the paleo diet, finding quick digesting pre-workout carbs is difficult with this one as your primary options are potatoes and fruit.

Additionally, this is also not a great diet for sedentary people, as they often substitute for the forbidden food groups with additional meat, nuts, and other high fat foods, making the diet inadvertently high in fat. And, while you can pretty easily stick to the diet for a whole 30 days, if you go back to binging your old foods to make up for all that lost time (which commonly happens after these kinds of ultra-restrictive diets), you can regain that lost weight, or even *more*! While this diet may be favored among people who are going to their high school reunions and want to look good, it is not designed to be a sustainable diet.

FAD DIETS WITH SOME MERIT

I'm not against most fad diets because they are popular, but because they are either bad for you, unsustainable, or both. A couple of them do have merit, however, and are worth considering as being suitable for certain situations.

The DASH Diet

DASH stands for Dietary Approaches to Stop Hypertension and focuses on reducing high blood pressure. This diet is good because it encourages you to eat vegetables, fruits, and whole grains. It includes fat-free or low-fat dairy products, fish, poultry, beans, and nuts, while limiting foods that are high in saturated fat (such as fatty meats and full-fat dairy products), and foods that are high in sodium or added sugars.

The Mediterranean Diet

This diet is based on the way several cultures—like those of Greece, Italy, and others from the Mediterranean region—that include whole grains, vegetables, legumes, fruits, nuts, and seeds. Olive oil is the main source of added fat. Processed foods, added sugar, and refined grains (i.e., anything made with white flour) are restricted or eliminated. Fish, seafood, dairy, and poultry are the main protein sources for this diet. Red meat and sweets are eaten only on occasion.

Both the DASH and the Mediterranean diets are pretty reasonable and well-aligned with my own diet and the principles I follow and recommend. However, both of these diets are more focused towards longevity than fitness, so the actual specifics of these two diets may not fit the needs of someone looking to achieve a better physique.

The "If It Fits Your Macros" (IIFYM) Diet

In the IIFYM diet, you track the total amount of fat, protein, and carbs (the "macros") that you eat each day. Using a macro calculator, you determine how much of each macro group you should eat per day to lose weight. Then you are allowed to consume those calories through whatever foods "fit" your macro requirements. This diet is more effective than calorie counting because it gives individually tailored macro limits based on the user's lifestyle and goals, while offering a lot of flexibility in what and when they eat to achieve it. This diet is the most similar in rationale and structure to the diet that I follow. However, for a beginner, I don't find IIFYM to be a great diet for two main reasons:

1. It tends to ignore calorie quality: Under this diet, if you stay within your macro "budget," *no food is off limits!* Unfortunately, this also means that all calories within a macro group are treated the same: carbs and fat from a snickers bar count the same toward your daily macro count as does avocado on high fiber toast. Carbs from gummy bears would be viewed the same as carbs from an apple. In short, this diet can still be pretty unhealthy if one chooses highly processed foods over whole foods that offer nutrients like fiber, vitamins, and minerals.

2. It also ignores macro balance within meals: as long as you meet your total protein, fat, and carb allotments for the day, it doesn't matter if the totals for each macro are split across the day or consumed within one meal. If you choose, you could eat all your daily carbs in one meal on this diet, which is a bad idea for those hoping to avoid blood sugar spikes and energy crashes.

The biggest takeaway from our review of these various diets is this: **don't cut out entire food groups**. Long-term scientific research show that people who eat a balanced omnivore diet with some but not excessive amounts of animal protein and high-quality fats have the best health outcomes and live the longest.

The second biggest takeaway concerns those who ask, "Isn't a calorie just a calorie, and aren't all calories the same?"

The answer is "yes," for weight loss, but food quality and macronutrient balance really do matter for energy levels, athletic performance, and long-term health! Let's turn now to how I put this all together to deliver the results I wanted while still having a balanced and enjoyable lifestyle.

"HOW I KEEP MY WEIGHT UNDER CONTROL"...OR LOW-STRESS DIET AND EXECUTION STRATEGIES

The "I Hate Diets" Diet

Dieting was always the hardest part of every competition prep period for me because it was the most regimented. Somehow, all of my coaches just assumed that I would be able to eat the same thing at the same time every day for my entire 4-month training cycle, and that I wouldn't be eating out with my friends or making plans for after work. It's no surprise that the athletes I knew who did the best with sticking to their training and their diet plans were the ones with the most predictable and least demanding work lives and personal schedules.

I, on the other hand, was single and trying to actively date for a good portion of my lifting tenure, so there was no way I was eating plain chicken and rice out of a Tupperware container every single night. Have you ever eaten healthy food on a date? No, you haven't, because you're trying to look lovable and fun, not robotic and uptight. I love eating and being able to do normal people things such as eating out and going on vacation whenever I like, even when I'm dieting. This often makes keeping my weight down challenging, and it definitely makes sticking with any fad diet pretty much impossible. But it shouldn't be impossible to balance a social life with the look and fitness level you want.

At the end of the day, what everyone here really wants to know is, "What's the best diet?" Well, *the best diet is the diet that you can actually stick to.* No fad diet or amount of science can do much for you if you can't stick to the routine for more than a few days. The best diet is well-balanced and practical enough to follow every day without feeling so hungry or inconvenienced that your quality of life is diminished.

I am hopeful that this diet can help you accomplish this. It's the diet I use to lose weight year-round before competition. It's optimized not for athletic performance, but primarily to maintain fitness while having a busy schedule and everyday life.

Weight Timing

Here are a couple of tips for keeping weight under control for those who rely on a scale to track their progress. Needless to say, a scale should keep us accountable, not make us obsessed!

- If you're trying to lose weight, aim for losing less than 1% of your body weight a week for sustainability. This makes the math easy. If you weigh 200 pounds, you should not aim to lose more than 2 pounds a week.

- Don't weigh yourself too often; body weight can fluctuate quite a bit day-to-day, depending on water retention. For consistency, weigh yourself at most once a week on the same day of the week, first thing in the morning.

Meal Timing

For a lot of people, diets don't work because they find themselves feeling too hungry throughout the day. Often this is caused by going too long in between meals (as in intermittent fasting), eating too little for some meals (as in any restrictive diet), or eating meals that lack proper macronutrient balance, particularly meals that are predominantly carbs (e.g., juice fasts, vegan, or other high-carb meals). Eating reasonably portioned meals that contain all macronutrient groups, spaced fairly evenly throughout the day, substantially helps to mitigate this.

Spacing meals evenly apart provides consistent energy to the body. While doing so won't change your metabolism, it will reduce energy crashes and keeps you from having major hunger pangs that cause you to go off the rails on your diet.

Here are some tips to optimizing meal timing according to your personal schedule:

- The exact time of day you eat each meal doesn't matter too much, but I recommend that you have three or four meals a day spaced fairly evenly apart depending on your schedule. For example, good spacing between meals might look like having breakfast at 8 a.m., lunch at noon, a snack at 3 p.m., and dinner at 7 p.m.

- If you have three meals instead of four, you can allow yourself one larger meal; this can be more emotionally satisfying, especially if it's a social meal (with friends or at an event).

- Large or heavy meals can lead to slumps in energy. Meals should not be too big, as we want every meal to be fully digested by the stomach before the next.

When your stomach is very full, your body needs to divert extra energy to digest all that food. This leads to you feeling tired and sleepy, which can be looked at as your body's natural signal that you've eaten too much.

- For those who exercise right before or after work, give yourself four meals for workout days, with two mini-meals that surround the workout. This will provide you with energy for your workout without you being too full to actually workout. A mini-meal can be something like cereal and yogurt, egg on toast, or a protein bar. If you can't eat before a workout because your stomach will feel upset doing vigorous activity, a protein shake may give you what you need without agitating the stomach.

- Time your workouts so that they are 2–3 hours after a meal. Ideally this meal should have carbs and protein but not too much fat so that it's fully digested by your stomach before your workout begins. Remember, fat requires a lot of energy and time to digest, so a very fatty meal could have you feeling sluggish for the next few hours. I prefer to have a very low-fat pre-workout meal so that I can work out closer to two hours after I eat. For me, this usually works out to a mid-day snack at 3 p.m. so that I can work out at 5 p.m. If your pre-workout meal has a full serving of added fat in it (more on this later), you may want to eat it closer to three hours prior to your workout to ensure that you have enough time to digest it.

- Your last meal should be at least two hours before bedtime. You'll have better sleep quality if you are not sleeping on a full stomach. If you're not able to eat your last meal until very close to when you'd like to go to sleep, try keeping this meal on the smaller and less fatty side, for the same reason.

"Does it matter when I eat? Do I have to eat every 3 hours, or something like that?"

You want to avoid going so long between meals that you'll be starving by the time you next eat. This is more likely to lead to overeating, and sometimes binging, for a couple of reasons. First, there will be a delayed response in your stomach between being full and your brain receiving the signal that you are full. And second, when you are ravenous, you are more likely to eat faster. Combine these two factors, and by the time you finally feel full, you'll have eaten a lot more calories than you would have otherwise.

(On a side note, I think this is why intermittent fasting is so popular: if you skip breakfast, you can achieve a 16-hour fast. Success! But then how are your energy levels going into lunch?)

If you're not a morning exercise person and you don't feel too hungry in the mornings, a good compromise to keep calories low and energy levels up is to have a protein shake for breakfast or skim milk in your coffee. When I'm on the road, I'll bring my own protein powder in a zip lock bag and throw half a scoop in my morning latte for a quick breakfast.

And just to bust a popular myth: eating smaller meals more frequently does NOT increase your metabolism. It just keeps you feeling energetic and satiated.

Leaning into Lean Protein

Not all animal protein is the same! Why is this? Because most meat and dairy are actually a combination of protein and fat. To make things even more confusing, the fat and protein percentages will also vary depending on what part of the animal the meat comes from. So, when picking your dietary protein, go for the lean meat. But what exactly counts as a "lean meat"?

According to the U.S. Department of Agriculture (the "USDA"), to be considered "lean," a 3.5 ounce serving of cooked beef must have less than 10 grams of total fat, 4.5 grams or less of saturated fat, and less than 95 mg of cholesterol. We will use this definition of less than 10 grams of total fat and 4.5 grams or less of saturated fat per serving for our definition of lean protein throughout this book.

So, for your meat and poultry choices, choose cuts that are labeled as at least 90% lean. If you can find meat or poultry that is 93-95% lean, that's even better. The most common lean poultry examples would be chicken breast or turkey breast. For beef, it would be beef round roast, round steak, and top sirloin. Most seafood found in Western diets are naturally lean, with mackerel, eel, salmon, and tuna belly being some common exceptions.

Eyeballing Your Food

Yes, before even tasting a food, we typically size it up with our eyes. Luckily, this also means that we can use our eyes to estimate the caloric value of foods without obsessing over a food calculator!

Rather than counting calories, I recommend following these approximate food portions using USDA serving sizes as visual markers:

1 serving lean protein (25 g = one deck of playing cards)

1 serving carb (15 g = 1 slice of bread)

1 serving fat (10 g = the size of the tip of your thumb, from the distal knuckle [the joint closest to the fingernail] to the tip)

Common Examples of Serving Sizes:

MACRONUTRIENT TYPE	SERVING SIZE	HEALTHY EXAMPLES
Protein	25 g	• 3 oz lean meat • 4 oz fish or shrimp • 2 whole eggs and 4 egg whites • 1½ cups nonfat Greek yogurt • 1 cup extra firm tofu
Carbohydrate	15 g	• 1/3 cup pasta or rice • 1 slice of bread • ½ cup sweet potato • 1/2 a banana • 1 small apple
Fat	10 g	• 1 tbsp butter or oil • 1 tbsp peanut butter • 15 almonds • 3 avocado slices
Fiber (technically, not a macronutrient)	1 cup	• broccoli • cauliflower • spinach • any kind of Lettuce • any color of bell pepper (not leafy or necessarily green, but very low calorie and healthy)

AN IMPORTANT TIP!

Make sure you know what an actual serving looks like! The modern diet is so carb heavy and fatty that most foods contain multiple servings of fat and carbs, and the average meal portion contains more than one serving of food. If you are trying to lose weight, you'll need to be mindful of not just what you eat, but of how much of it you are eating.

And Now, The Actual Diet

[DISCLAIMER: *If you have any food allergies or intolerances, in accordance with the disclaimer at the beginning of this book, you should consult with a qualified doctor, nutritionist, or other healthcare provider before making any substantial changes to your diet.*]

Let's be real, no one wants to weigh their food or count calories, and very few people are happy about using food calculators to tabulate every portion of every meal down to the last drop of oil. So how do we make things simpler?

Think 1:2:1

I like to have a 1:2:1 protein/carb/fat ratio for my meals. Each of my daily meals then works out to something like:

> 1 serving lean protein + 2 servings carb + 1 serving fat + 1 cup of leafy greens (raw or cooked, but with no added fat)

Let's say you are a starting or recreational athlete who wants to lose weight at a reasonable rate, while strength training for three one-hour sessions a week along with two hours a week of moderate cardio a week. For the easiest math, I would recommend the following:

consume 80% your bodyweight in lbs. in total grams of protein a day

This works out conveniently because if you choose your bodyweight in pounds as the number of total grams of carbs you can consume each day, you can have one serving of fat with each of your three or four meals and still be within a healthy calorie range for weight loss.

IMPORTANT STRENGTH TRAINING TIP

If you are going to add strength training to your fitness regimen, you will need to eat *more* protein, that is, enough to repair and grow your muscles. The Academy of Nutrition and Dietetics and the American College of Sports Medicine both recommend that athletes eat 1.2 to 2 grams of protein per kilogram (2.2 lb.) of body weight— this is anywhere from 55–90% of your body weight in pounds, in grams of protein. The percentage should increase the more intense and often your strength training workouts are, so someone primarily doing cardio would use closer to 55% of their bodyweight while an avid lifter would be closer to 90%.

Using myself as an example, the daily protein requirement for a 125 lb. lightly-active adult woman is 125 x 80% = 100 g, which divides very easily into 25 g per meal across four meals:

MEAL 1	25 g
MEAL 2	25 g
MEAL 3	25 g
MEAL 4	25 g
TOTAL MEALS	Total Protein = 100 g
TOTAL CALORIES	400 calories

Each gram of protein is 4 calories, as I need 400 calories of protein daily.

My daily carbs would be 125 g, which we can round to 30 g per meal. Keep in mind that's 15 g x 2 portions from the 1:2:1 ratio:

MEAL 1	30 g
MEAL 2	30 g
MEAL 3	30 g
MEAL 4	30 g
TOTAL MEALS	Total Carbs = 125g, rounded to 120g for easier math
TOTAL CALORIES	480 calories

Each gram of carbohydrate is 4 calories, as I also need 400 calories of carbs daily.

This actually matches 1 USDA serving size of protein and 2 servings of carbs per meal. The math may not work out as conveniently at every weight, but the goal here is simply to estimate your protein and carb targets per day.

Now let's turn to total fat, a subject that begins with an important caveat: most of the protein that you consume will also have some fat, so here we are talking about added fat *outside* of your protein. I find that the math works out the easiest if I allow myself one serving of added fat per meal, so that I'm eating the same servings of fat per meal as I am protein.

In order to factor in this caveat, we must double the calculation for fat.

MEAL 1	10 g (from protein) + 10 g (additional source) = 20 g
MEAL 2	10 g (from protein) + 10 g (additional source) = 20 g
MEAL 3	10 g (from protein) + 10 g (additional source) = 20 g
MEAL 4	10 g (from protein) + 10 g (additional source) = 20 g
TOTAL MEALS	Total Fat = 80 g
TOTAL CALORIES	800 calories

Each gram of fat is 9 calories, but rounding it up for easier math we'll call it 10 calories, which is how I get to my 800 calories of fat per day.

When we add all the macronutrients together, this is what we get for me:

PROTEIN	CARBS	FATS	TOTAL CALORIES
400	480	800	1680

Given my body's daily caloric needs, consuming this total number of calories daily puts me at a small caloric deficit. Since my body needs 1,800 to 2,100 calories to maintain my weight, 1,680 calories means that I'm on track to lose ½ to 1 pound per week!

If you've kept up with the math, you'll also know that this means I get a total of 4 servings of protein, 8 servings of carbs, and 4 servings of added fat every day. I find this daily total to be more helpful than a total calorie count because this makes it easy to move a serving of carbs or fat to another meal whenever I want to deviate from my 1:2:1 ratio for a meal or two while still maintaining my total daily calorie goal.

One Size Does *Not* Fit All—Figuring Out How Many Calories *Your* Body Burns

Here's the reality: the bigger you are, the more calories you burn throughout the day. A 6'2" person burns more calories than a 5'4" person of similar build because their larger body needs more energy to sustain their system.

Aside from height, calories are also affected by how active you are, your age, your sex, and how much muscle you have as well as your *current* weight.

I'll demonstrate below using myself, a 125 lb. woman, as an example. For the male example, we will use a 200 lb. man.

How To Calculate Your Metabolism With BMR

Your Basal Metabolic Rate (BMR) is how many calories you need just to sustain your body and keep you alive. It is the baseline number from which our metabolism is calculated. There are many scientifically validated BMR equations, but one of the most commonly used—which we will use here—is the Mifflin-St. Jeor Equation:

MEN	(10 × weight in kg) + (6.25 × height in cm) − (5 × age in years) + 5
WOMEN	(10 × weight in kg) + (6.25 × height in cm) − (5 × age in years) − 161

For example, if a man is 200 lbs. (which converts to 90.7 kg), and he is 6 feet tall (which converts to about 183 cm), and he is 30 years old, then the math would look like this:

(10 x 90.7) + (6.25 x 183) − (5 x 30) + 5
BMR = 907 + 1143.8 − 150 + 5 = 1,905.8 calories BMR

Now let's calculate for a woman who is 125 lbs. (which converts to 56.7 kg), and who is 5'4" (which converts to 162.5 cm), and who is 30 years old; for this woman, the math would look like this:

(10 x 56.7) + (6.25 x 162.5) − (5 x 30) - 161
BMR = 567 + 1015.6 - 150 − 161 = 1271.6 calories BMR

Here's a set of convenient blank template so you can determine your own numbers:

Men:

Converting from pounds to kilograms:
_____ lbs. ÷ 2.2 = _____ kg

Converting from inches to centimeters:
_____ in. x 2.54 = _____ cm

BMR = (10 x _____kg) + (6.25 x _____cm) −
(5 x _____ [your age]) + 5 = _____ calories BMR

Women:

Converting from pounds to kilograms:
_____ lbs. ÷ 2.2 = _____ kg

Converting from inches to centimeters:
_____ in. x 2.54 = _____ cm

BMR = (10 x _____kg) + (6.25 x _____cm) −
(5 x _____ [your age]) − 30 = _____ calories BMR

One very interesting thing to note about this equation, as well as all of the other BMR equations, is that for a male-female pair of the exact same weight, height, and age, the man will always have a higher BMR than the woman! Not fair!

With more natural muscle mass, men are thermogenically less efficient than women, and their bodies generate more heat, giving them a higher basal metabolic rate (BMR) than women when controlling for age, height, and weight. Remember, your BMR is how many calories you need just to sustain your body and stay alive.

Now you might think, "Wait a minute...I'm pretty active, so shouldn't I have a higher BMR? Doesn't muscle burn more calories, and all that?"

Keep in mind that even someone who doesn't exercise, per se, still moves around somewhat, thereby using more energy daily than what their BMR indicates is required for the basic bodily functions that keeps them alive. In practice, it therefore makes sense to use a multiplying factor to make adjustments to your BMR to better estimate your actual daily calorie maintenance level.

To determine a number closer to your actual BMR, multiply your BMR from the equation by the following factors, based on your physical activity:

ACTIVITY LEVEL	MULTIPLYING FACTOR
Sedentary (no exercise)	X 1.2
Lightly Active (light exercise 1–3 days/week)	X 1.375
Moderately Active (exercise 3–5 days/week)	X 1.55
Very Active (exercises every day or physically active job)	X 1.9

If you don't do any formal exercise but have a job or lifestyle that requires a lot of physical activity, you can also approximate your activity level using your step count:

- Fewer than 1,000 steps a day is Sedentary.

- 1,000 to 10,000 steps or about 4 miles a day is Lightly Active.

- 10,000 to 23,000 steps or 4 to 10 miles a day is considered Moderately Active.

- More than 23,000 steps or 10 miles a day is Very Active.

Using the above example of the 30-year-old 125 lb. woman with a BMR of 1,272 calories (rounding up!), if she is sedentary, she will actually burn 1,526 calories, which is a huge difference. But if she is lightly active, she will burn 1,748 which is even of a difference!

How to Passively Burn More Calories

One more thing about BMR calculators before we end this section: BMR is largely influenced by a person's muscle mass. Muscle uses more energy than fat at rest. Therefore, the more muscle you have, the higher your metabolism is relative to those your exact same weight! If two people are the same age, height, gender and the exact same weight, the person with more muscle will have the higher metabolism. Not that you needed a reason to lift weights before, but if you did, this would be it!

The estimated increase in metabolism may not seem like much; scientists have measured that a pound of muscle burns 6–7 more calories per day than a pound of fat. If you have three extra pounds of muscle, your body will burn about an additional 150 calories each week automatically, making it that much easier to get to your weight goals.

More importantly, extra muscle mass is not accounted for in the BMR equations, so no need to get too hung up on exact BMR numbers. Think of extra muscle on your body like extra credit and remember that your BMR calculation might vary from your actual metabolism as you get into better shape.

Since You Know the Rules, You can Choose When to Bend Them

Even following the above recommendations, your body might require additional adjustments based on your ongoing weight loss progress AND how you are actually feeling.

If you find yourself always feeling hungry or losing weight too fast (see earlier when I recommend losing less than 1% of your total bodyweight weekly), I would add in an extra serving of protein each day if you're aiming for muscle gain, or an extra serving of carbs before your workout if you feel that you need more energy for your workouts. Otherwise, if you're mainly aiming to look good, you can add a serving per day of any macronutrient group whenever you'd most like.

If you want to lose weight faster and don't mind compromising your workout quality or muscle composition, you can remove one serving of carbs from a meal or two, but avoid removing carbs from meals right before or right after your workout. For the rest of that day's meals, you should still aim to have all three macronutrient groups to avoid any type of energy crash.

You can also make two meals into one snack and one slightly bigger meal (just try to maintain some multiplier of your ratio for both meals), or consolidate two meals for the big meal when doing three meals.

Snacks can be carb-free if they aren't immediately before or after a workout (which is when you'll want and need them the most).

Why Leafy Greens are the "Best Cheat" for Your Diet

Add leafy greens to *every* meal for added fiber, nutrition, and fullness. These types of vegetables—which take up space in your stomach, yet are low in calories—help prevent you from eating higher calorie foods. They also contain fiber, which keeps you fuller longer and helps your digestion and elimination.

Greens may be cooked however you like as long as there's no added fat, which means baking, steaming, or sautéing using nonfat cooking spray. Unfortunately, if you add or dip your greens in butter for flavor, that adds in calories, which defeats the purpose of eating the greens in the first place. So best to steer clear of the butter.

If you want to feel fuller faster (and thus eat less), *eat your leafy greens first* before eating the rest of your meal. It's perfectly understandable if you don't want to eat broccoli with your breakfast, so if you don't want to eat leafy greens with your first meal of the day, that's fine. Instead, for this meal's serving of carbs, aim to have a high-fiber carb such as high-fiber toast. Similarly, you can also pick carbs that are higher in fiber for your other meals to supplement the vegetables in each meal. A popular choice for a high-fiber carb is the sweet potato, not only because is it high in fiber, but because it contains many other vitamins and nutrients.

How to Keep your Fat Intake Under Control

For fats, try to stick to good fats (unsaturated fats). Unsaturated fats in reasonable amounts are believed to improve blood cholesterol levels, ease inflammation, stabilize heart rhythms, and be good for brain and mental health. Saturated fats are fine in low amounts, but too much can be bad for your heart.

The above eating plan assumes that all food is cooked in little to no butter or oil. I cook my meals using fat-free cooking spray when dieting because even a small amount of cooking oil adds a lot of fat to your meal. However, if you really want to fry your meal in oil or butter, that should count as the total fat for that meal.

Do you remember during our discussion of 1:2:1 when we doubled the fat amount in our calorie calculation to accommodate the fat that comes with protein? Even with doubling the fat amount, those calculations are estimated assuming that you are eating a lean protein as your protein choice for every meal.

This mostly applies to meat such as poultry, pork, and beef, as well as dairy. Seafood is naturally lean with a few exceptions, and seed protein cannot be made lean. This means that you'll have to assume your protein choice has an extra serving of fat per serving on most meat or dairy not labeled "lean" or "nonfat."

Here are some portions of meat with a higher fat content. You need to factor in extra fat into these particular foods:

- Dairy products—cheese that's not labeled "light," "low-fat," or "nonfat"

- Steak

- Chicken thighs or drumsticks

- Tuna belly

Some of you might want to say, "But wait! Isn't chicken supposed to be a healthy protein!" In fact, mostly it is! However, many people don't realize that not all parts of an animal are equally lean. While a chicken breast is indeed one of the best sources of protein, a chicken thigh has more fat in it. And if you prepare it fried, there's even more fat because of how it's cooked.

When you consume these foods, mentally calculate them as "one protein + one additional fat." Again, this doesn't mean avoiding foods. It just means that you should be aware that it's the fat that provides the flavor, so naturally we all want more flavor in our food. So we have to watch it.

Example Meals

Let's turn to some example meal plan to see what it looks like when we put it all together. Here, then, are some of my sample meals for staying in shape when not in competition prep:

> [NOTE: *An asterisk (*) denotes where I might cut one serving of carbs if I was trying to lose more weight more aggressively. A double asterisk (**) denotes where I removed a serving of fat. If I'm not trying to aggressively diet, I can add a second serving of added fat to any of the three other meals to hit my daily 4:8:4 serving total.]*

BREAKFAST:

- 1 egg + 2 egg whites scramble with 1 serving of cheese on 2 slices of wheat toast*, coffee with a little nonfat milk (1 serving of protein, 2 of carbs, 1 of added fat)

LUNCH:

- 3 oz of chicken + 1 serving cauliflower + 1 serving avocado + ⅔ cup of rice (1 serving of protein, 2 of carbs, 1 of added fat)

PRE-WORKOUT MEAL**:

- Nonfat Greek yogurt + 2 servings of low-fat cereal like Cinnamon Toast Crunch (1 serving of protein, 2 of carbs, and no added fats so the food digests in time for working out)

DINNER:

- 4 oz of fish + 1 serving broccoli + 1 serving avocado + ⅔ cup of rice (1 serving of protein, 2 of carbs, 1 of added fat)

Here are some sample meals for when I'm traveling:

BREAKFAST ON THE GO:

- Coffee with 2 tbsps. nonfat milk, a scoop of protein powder, and Splenda (1 serving of protein, moving the carbs and fats to the next meal for a bigger lunch)

LUNCH FROM A RESTAURANT:

- Turkey avocado sandwich with no mayo + a salad with no dressing + 1 small cookie or a bag of chips (1 serving of protein, 4 of carbs, 2 of added fat)

DINNER FROM A RESTAURANT (combine the food servings from the pre-workout meal and dinner):

- Grilled seafood (usually 8 oz) with veggies (there's always some sauce or added fat) + some complimentary bread* (2 servings of protein, 2 of carbs, 1 of added fat)

Followed by whatever workout I can squeeze in at the hotel gym.

"Wait! This is Supposedly Easy and Simple; I Need Easier and Simpler Than This!"

If you don't want to think about weighing food or planning your meals, here are some of the simplest things you can do to lose weight in a balanced and healthy way. In fact, if you don't want to do anything else recommended in this book, at the very least, consider following the suggestions in the list below. If you do so, you will almost certainly lose weight, as the amount of calorie-dense food available to you will be so greatly reduced that your daily calorie intake will likely fall of its own accord:

- **Eat less fatty cuts of meat**; choose grilled fish and chicken breast.

- **Avoid milk fats** (pick nonfat milk and yogurt) and cheese.

- **Avoid fats, both as a cooking method or a sauce.** When eating out, foods that are boiled, steamed, baked, or braised will have less added fat than other cooking methods. **Especially avoid deep fried foods** as they have too many added calories; many foods absorb oil very well and deep frying can *triple* the amount of calories in a food. Also, science is finding that deep fried foods and trans fats increase the risk of heart disease, cancer, and diabetes. Similarly, anything breaded and fried is going to be a calorie bomb since the breading absorbs oil amazingly well.

- **Reduce your carb consumption** by swapping carbs with leafy greens as much as possible.

- **Don't drink your calories.** You won't feel full and the instant surge in blood sugar will lead to an energy crash; remember, this is why juice fasts are a terrible idea. For similar reasons, avoid alcohol; not only is it empty calories, but in the short-term, it increases your appetite (who hasn't had post-drinking food binge?). It also negatively impacts your hormones in a way that increases fat storage (especially belly fat), as well as decreases athletic performance.

- **Avoid ultra-processed foods.** What's an ultra-processed food? Foods with added ingredients that act as stabilizers, preservatives, or texturizes (e.g., Doritos, hot dogs, Oreos, and nearly all fast food). An easy way to tell if a food is ultra-processed is whether or not it can be made in a home kitchen, either because it contains chemicals that normal people can't get, or requires production methods that a normal kitchen wouldn't have. It has been found that ultra-processed foods alter the satiety process and blood sugar response of the body in a way that causes you to eat more. Also, taking in large amounts of processed food can increase the risk of diabetes, heart disease, and cerebrovascular diseases.

- **It's best to avoid these foods** that we tend to think are diet friendly, but actually aren't:

  - *Salad dressing, sandwich spreads like aioli or mayonnaise, and nut butters like peanut butter*, which are very fatty and thus calorie dense. Also, almost nobody eats just one serving at a time of these; it's typically three or more!

  - *Barbecue sauce* (or other sweet sauces like *teriyaki*). These sauces are pure sugar, and everyone always uses more than one serving, which means lots of added calories.

♦ *Açaí bowls and smoothies.* These "healthy drinks" are actually loaded with carbs, full of calories, and can cause large blood sugar spike if consumed on their own.

♦ *Dried fruit.* Dried fruit has all the fiber and nutrients of regular fruit. As such, it is actually somewhat healthy. The problem is, without the water, it's hard to feel full from eating dried fruit, and it becomes very easy to eat a lot of it. You probably couldn't eat 5 apricots in one sitting, but you could easily eat 5 dried apricots. Fruit is already high in sugar. Dried fruit contains 3 to 4 times the amount of sugar and calories per weight compared to its undried equivalent!

♦ *Granola.* Granola is loaded with both carbs and fats; after all, it is just cereal (carbs) mixed with sugar (more carbs), and then fat to hold it together. Calorically, granola is almost the same as eating crumbled up cookies (and I'd much rather have the cookies). Obviously, if we're avoiding granola, the same goes for granola bars and trail mixes!

How to Make this Diet Work When Eating Out

The truth of the matter is that dieting can be pretty difficult when you are going out to eat. Many of us dine out multiple times a week, so for this diet to succeed, it's important to have a strategy for how to eat out without eating more than you want to.

Things to keep in mind when eating out:

• Everything at a restaurant is prepared with added fat, even things you normally would not add fat to (like steamed vegetables). Assume your one serving of fat for this meal is already used in the food preparation method.

- All cuts of meat are fattier at a restaurant than what you would prepare at home. This is because it makes the food cheaper and tastier. Choose seafood as your protein as the fat content in the protein will not differ (although the cooking method might add fat).

- All restaurant sauces have added sugar and/or fat. You can be sure that your neighborhood Italian restaurant is pumping its marinara full of olive oil and sugar to make it extra tasty. If you can, get all dressings and sauces on the side and eat as little of it as you can. If you are feeling extra virtuous, ask for all of your dishes sauce-free.

- At this point, you're aware that all mayos, spreads, and aiolis are added fat. But also, restaurants use more than one serving of each when preparing food. Sure, one tablespoon of mayo in a sandwich tastes good, but three servings? Three servings makes a sandwich taste great! And now you've eaten almost all your added fat for the day. Keep any fatty condiment to a bare minimum.

- Sadly, the same rule also applies to cheese. Avoid adding cheese to sandwiches or burgers when eating out because much like with mayo, restaurants will usually exceed one serving when adding this.

What about Snacks?
Do I Have to Avoid Them Completely?

Snacks with some amount of protein in them tend to have the biggest bang-per-calorie-buck when it comes to satiety.

Some good examples would include sugar-free nonfat yogurt, protein bars, or nuts. Keep in mind that for nuts, the fat-to-protein ratio is relatively high, so don't go too crazy on the serving size. Avoid meat jerky unless it's nitrate-free (another example of an ultra-processed food).

Eating Differently If You Are Sporty or Actively Training for a Sport

If you're implementing this diet alongside training for a sport or athletic event, you may find that you want to modify the macronutrient ratios for the specific goals of your sport. For weightlifting and other strength focused sports, you might benefit from a higher protein, medium carb, and lower fat daily macronutrient ratio. For endurance, you might want to employ a higher carb, medium protein, and lower fat ratio. As you get more specialized in your athletic training, the ratios will be more specific to your goals and meal timing, so these are just some general guidelines.

Also, keep in mind that weight loss can definitely compromise strength and athletic performance, so if you're trying to diet while training for a sport or an athletic event, I'd recommend hiring a specialized diet coach. The ins and outs of sports training while in a caloric deficit can be pretty nuanced, and you wouldn't want some random stranger giving you bad advice and compromising your performance.

"Do I Have to Eat Like This All The Time?"

No, not all the time, but most of the time. Personally, I like having a more caloric "cheat meal" twice a week. I try to space these out so they are at least two days apart.

To keep myself motivated, I used to tell myself that if I stuck to my diet, I could have a cheat meal with friends Thursday night and then again on Saturday. There is a positive psychological aspect to this where you don't feel like you're missing out on life or starving all the time. However, try not to go too crazy during these cheat meals: it's a slippery slope that can lead to undoing the calorie deficit you already worked so hard to attain during the week.

So, as much as you can help it, try not to eat more than double the amount of food that you would for your regular meal in this meal. For example, I would aim to eat less than 2 servings of protein + 4 servings of carbs + 2 servings of fats for a cheat meal.

If you mess up on this every so often, don't be too hard on yourself. Unless you're a heartless robot, everyone has moments where they're bad at self-control. Consistency does not mean never messing up; it means always being willing to try again and try your best! The most important thing is adhering to the diet as much as you can. Even if you have a bad meal, you're still doing much better in the grand scheme of things, so don't give up. Diets aren't all or nothing; even if you follow only 80% of this diet, you can still get great results!

PART 2

EXERCISE AND MOVEMENT

Before we dive into the actual exercises, let's address some common workout myths I hear all too often:

> *"I don't have hours a day to dedicate to getting in shape."*

Okay, so this is your reminder that for weight loss to be both successful and sustainable, you need to drop the "all or nothing" mentality. You don't need to follow every piece of advice in this book perfectly every day to see positive changes, but you do need to do *something*. Remember, even just 20 minutes of intense cardio, three times a week is enough to improve your fitness. If you're busy, your best bet is to do as much of a high intensity workout as you can, even if you can't do as much of it as you want. Doing even just a little bit of exercise is infinitely better than doing none at all.

> *"But I just want a six pack."*

Contrary to popular belief, "spot workouts" such as doing sit-ups or other exercises that only target your abs will not burn belly fat or get you six-pack abs. You can make an individual muscle bigger, but there's no natural way to reduce fat from just one region of the body. The reality is that to lose belly fat, you simply have to lose fat in general. Then you'll see abs!

"Muscle makes women bulky."

It is typically quite hard for a female to get significantly more muscular while both dieting and lifting weights (trust me, I've tried!). You'd have to dedicate a lot of effort to eating more to become bulky from lifting just 3 hours a week. Also, some muscle tone in the thighs and arms emphasize the curvature of the limb and make your limbs actually appear longer and leaner (and less saggy!).

Another side benefit of lifting weights is that building muscle helps you ongoingly burn more calories, since muscle uses calories even when you are not exercising. Cardio only burns calories in the moment, whereas strength training can increase your metabolism for the next few days as your body will need to use calories to repair the muscles and other tissues used during the workout.

"But I just wanna tone."

What most people consider toned—being slim with nice curves—is just a combination of losing fat while building some muscle at the same time. If you just lose the fat without adding any muscle, you'll look like a stick.

"Chest workouts make women flat chested."

A lot of women specifically do not want to work out their upper bodies because they worry that their breasts will turn into flat chiseled pecs alongside gigantic, rounded shoulders. First of all, breasts are made of fat. Weight loss involves fat reduction. Therefore, any successful diet will decrease your breast size, whether or not any chest exercises are involved.

Secondly, you would have to bench press an extreme amount of weight consistently for this to happen—far beyond what this book recommends—so your boobs are probably safe. In fact, slightly increasing the size of the pec muscles under your breasts *does* give your breasts a fuller volume and make them a little perkier! However, if poppin' pecs are not something that you are interested in, go ahead and swap the bench press exercises in this book's example workouts for shoulder presses or something similar.

CARDIO

"Cardio"—the colloquial term for cardiovascular workouts—gets its own section here because of the many myths and unfounded ideas associated with it. Cardio workouts focus on exercising with a sustained elevated heart rate following the belief that this is the most effective kind of workout. This assumption makes sense: whenever we look at cyclists, sprinters, soccer players, or swimmers, they are visual examples of lean bodies with anatomical definition.

Many people, therefore, seem to think that losing weight and looking good means hours on the treadmill. Luckily for us, there are other, and in my opinion, *better* ways to get in shape than this. Personally, I have always hated doing cardio, especially running. There is no worse feeling than huffing and puffing while being uncomfortable and sweaty as your body slowly overheats.

Not only are long bouts of high intensity cardio unpleasurable for many, but cardio will *not* give you sexy curves or muscle. Yes, it does burn a lot of calories, so it can help you get skinnier, but not skinnier in a way that I personally find sexy. I lost the most weight and looked what I thought was the best through heavy weightlifting, whether it was bodybuilding or powerlifting. I also felt less sweaty and exhausted after these workouts compared to running. You should do at least *some* cardio as it is beneficial for your heart and general health, but you don't need to do hours upon hours of it to reap substantial benefits.

If you do happen to *love* cardio, and you are physically (and emotionally!) capable of handling it, just one total hour of intense cardio a week will give you a range of general health benefits. The ideal intensity is where it is challenging to carry on a conversation but not so hard that you aren't able to say a few words during the activity. You can break the hour up into two or three shorter sessions across the week if that helps you complete the task.

If vigorous cardio is not something that you feel that you can do, you can spend more time with low-impact exercises like brisk walking or riding an exercise bike. Aim for 90 minutes a week with low impact cardio when doing this alongside lifting, or you can increase it if it's your sole exercise for the week.

You can also increase calorie burn via non-exercise movement. You can take the stairs instead of the elevator. If you commute via train or bus, exit one stop earlier and walk the rest of the way. If it's safe to do so, take a 20-minute walk around the block every night after dinner. If you have a smartwatch or phone with a pedometer feature, you can also just aim to increase your footsteps by 1,000–2,000 steps a day and increase your pace accordingly.

I know some people who pace around their house or office every few hours as a way to do this. I even had one colleague who used to vigorously jump up and down on the lab floor every few hours to lose weight. It may look funny, but I'm all for doing whatever works for you. I personally purchased Amazon's cheapest recumbent bike and placed it in front of my TV because slow stationary biking is a lot less boring while you're binge-watching trash TV. Rebounding, or bouncing on a high-quality mini-trampoline or rebounder, is also something you can do at home in front of the TV.

THE WORKOUT SECTION, OR "BARE MINIMUM WEEKLY WORKOUTS TO LOOK GOOD NAKED"

The best workout is the one that fits your lifestyle and that you will actually do. Therefore, a variety of different plans are provided that you can use to jumpstart your progress. With that said, I'll also offer my own recommendations as to what I found most effective as well as different ways to get to the same goal.

"How often should I work out?"

Three to four one-hour strength training sessions per week are adequate for most people. These workouts should be supplemented with some sort of cardio, either after your workout or on separate days.

For beginners, start with 2–3 lifting sessions a week (one upper body and one lower body if doing only two sessions a week) and increase as your level of fitness improves. Do cardio on your other workout days.

Also, muscle needs time to heal (and grow) properly. The more intense the workout is for a particular muscle, the longer that muscle needs to heal. Deadlifts are fairly taxing on the back, so I wouldn't recommend doing them more than once a week. Similarly, it's best not to squat more than two times a week. If you are only doing one exercise for a given muscle group per workout (e.g., a few sets of a single abs or triceps exercise), you can do this fairly often per week. For the general fitness workouts below, if you are hitting a double-digit number of total sets like 12 or 16 across the entire workout, it'd be best to give at least three days before working out the same muscle group again.

For all exercises, I suggest 3 or 4 sets of 8–10 reps at a slightly challenging weight. For all working sets (those done after the warm-up sets, as explained below), rest 2 minutes between sets, or 3 minutes between if the set feels particularly challenging or tiring.

General Advice on the Exercises and How to Perform Them

Most of the exercises recommended in this book are fairly common ones that most people have heard of. There is a good reason for this—because they work! Chances are, you have done at least some of these exercises before or have some understanding of what they should look like. You can find many detailed tutorials on how to perform any of these movements online; I would even suggest that you look up a video tutorial for each movement on a website like Bodybuilding.com before trying it yourself in the gym as a video will provide far more clarity than text explanations can. Here I'll provide some additional details on the different ways each movement can be performed while suggesting alternative exercises that suit your needs and circumstances and will similarly benefit you. Also, before you read the exercise tutorials, please keep in mind the following pointers:

- When instructed to "squeeze" a muscle during a movement, what this really means is to contract that muscle as much as you can. Typically, this will feel like the sensation that the muscle is squeezing itself, hence the term.

- For certain movements, having a slow, controlled release of the movement— approximately 2–4 seconds in duration—will accentuate strength building. The negative, or "release," portion of the movement is known as the "eccentric" phase of a lift, and we will refer to it as such from here on out. The exercises where a slow eccentric counts the most have been noted!

- The workouts are generically structured so that you can make use of whatever kind of equipment you have access to, whether it's dumbbells, barbells, or kettlebells. However, if you're a beginner, my order of equipment preference for you would be first dumbbells, then barbells, then kettlebells. Dumbbells tend to be more beginner friendly since they require you to use less total body parts for stabilization, and since each dumbbell moves independent of the other, they can help improve your form and correct muscle imbalances. Relative to dumbbells, barbells and kettlebells tend to cause more injuries for new lifters as proper technique is less intuitive for these movements.

- To strengthen your muscles in different ranges of motion and address any weak points, change up and vary the exercises from time to time. If you are trying to get stronger at a specific lift, such as the squat, I would perform that lift consistently every week until I achieved my desired strength result, but at the same time vary some of the other lifts within that workout each week.

- For all bold font exercises that use equipment like dumbbells, barbells, or kettlebells, start with two lighter warmup sets, increasing the weight after both sets, before then starting the "working set." The warmup sets should not count towards that exercise's sets or repetitions count.

- For each exercise's main working set, you'll want to pick a weight that is challenging but not impossible: pick a weight at which you can do every rep with good form, but with the last two reps being somewhat difficult. A good gauge for the right amount of difficulty is that you will need to struggle a little to complete the last two reps of the set, and the speed of these two reps will be noticeably less than the previous reps. When you get strong enough to do all reps at that weight without any difficulty, add about 2.5% more weight or whatever is the smallest increment of weight you can add to come up with your new working weight.

- The advice here is not specific to any particular body type, so generic instructions like "slight but not excessive rounding of the back" will differ in exactly how they apply to different people. If you experience difficulty in determining what's meant here and you're unsure of your form, I would recommend considering going through the exercises and techniques in question at least a few times with a qualified exercise coach or trainer, either remotely or in-person, until you get the hang of it.

- Along these same lines, the exercise pointers being given here are not sport-specific and are written generically to include beginners. As you grow more accustomed to the lifts or get more specific in your training, you may want to vary the technique slightly to accommodate your new circumstances. For example, an absolute beginner to lifting may only have enough strength or flexibility to perform squats in a certain way. However, as their supportive muscles get stronger and more flexible, they may find that they can implement helpful modifications to their original stance to improve squat efficiency that were not possible before.

STAYING IN SHAPE WHILE ON THE ROAD (AGAIN)

When traveling, if possible, try to pick a hotel with a gym. This is your best chance at squeezing in some sort of workout during your travels. Be realistic: you're just not going to take two hours out of your workday or vacation time to drive to a local gym for a workout. Some hotel gyms only have cardio machines. In these situations, just do the best you can. Do extra cardio until you have access to a gym again or do the bodyweight workout described below in the hotel gym or your hotel room as you have time; you can even break it up and do one exercise at a time if that's all you can squeeze in.

THE EXERCISES

The exercises are categorized and listed according to the following body regions:

- Upper Body (above the waist)
- Lower Body (below the waist)
- Back
- Abdominals
- Whole Body

These will be the building blocks for the workout routines that are considered later. They've been listed together in this way because there are multiple ways to work out different regions of the body. Under each exercise are my personal tips to make the most of the motion you're undertaking (and your time).

UPPER BODY

BENCH PRESS—While lying on a bench, push the weight away from your body and return the weight to its original position.

- This can be performed with a barbell or a dumbbell.
- Muscle group(s) worked: Mostly chest and triceps. Some shoulders.
- Variation:
  - *Incline Bench Press*—An angled bench press where your head is above your torso, increasing the focus on upper chest and shoulders.

BICEPS CURL—The weight is lifted towards your shoulder, bending at the elbow with palms facing the ceiling, followed by lowering the weight back to its original position.

- This can be performed with a barbell or a dumbbell.
- Muscle group(s) worked: Biceps.
- Variations:
    - *Hammer Curl*—The weight is held with your palms facing inward toward your body instead of toward the ceiling, with your arm and weight resembling a hammer.
    - *Seated Concentration Curl*—Sitting on a bench, the back of your arm rests against your inner thigh, making the arm more stable and focusing the bicep's contraction.

- Pointers: Squeeze your biceps at the top of the movement. For extra strength building, release the curl slowly for a 3-second count.

LATERAL RAISE—With palms facing the body, raise the weight until it is at shoulder height. If you raise both weights at once, your body forms a "T."

- This can be performed with dumbbells while standing or seated.
- Muscle group(s) worked: Front and side shoulders.
- The muscles worked don't vary too much between standing or seated, but when performing this lift while standing, be mindful not to swing your upper body in an attempt to assist your arms with the lift.
- Pointer: To prevent swinging, raise the weight slowly then hold it at the top of the movement for a full second.

PUSH-UPS—While lying on the floor, press your bodyweight up by straightening your arms.

- Muscle group(s) worked: Triceps and chest.
- Variations:
  - *Push-Up From Knees*—A beginner-friendly variant that reduces the amount of bodyweight to lift off the floor.
  - *Incline Push-Up*—An incline push-up is standard push-up performed with your upper body elevated; typically, your hands are placed on a bench or a raised surface. This is a great progression for anyone who finds push-ups from the knees very easy but can't quite perform a full push-up. The higher the incline, the more assistance you have in the movement, and the less of your bodyweight you'll effectively lift.

- Pointer: Keep your stomach tight with all push-ups so that your body maintains a straight line during the movement.

REAR DELT FLY: While the upper body is bent at the waist until your back is nearly parallel to the floor, both arms are raised to shoulder height with your palms facing the ground.

- This can be performed with dumbbells while standing or seated.
- Muscle group(s) worked: Rear shoulders.
- When comparing sitting and standing, there's little variation in the way that the muscles are worked. For either sitting or standing, be mindful not to swing your upper body to assist you with the lift. To prevent excessive swinging, try performing these seated while bent over, or you can rest your chest on a bench.

SHOULDER PRESS—With the upper body in a fully vertical position, press the weight from shoulder level until it is vertically overhead, then return it to its original position.

- This can be performed with a barbell or dumbbells, while standing or seated
- Muscle group(s) worked:
  - Seated—Mostly shoulders. Some triceps.
  - Standing—Mostly shoulders, some triceps, some upper back.

- Variation:
  - *Arnold Press*—The Arnold press (named after bodybuilding great and former California governor Arnold Schwarzenegger) starts with your palms facing your body and your upper arm close to the front of your body. Unlike the shoulder press, your palms will be in front of your face as you begin the press. As you press, rotate the dumbbells away for your centerline until your palms are facing forward like a standard dumbbell press. The rotation of the dumbbells from the front of your body to the side will build the side and back portion of your shoulders in addition to the front portion of the shoulders that already get strengthened during the standard shoulder press.

- Pointers: You can be seated or standing for shoulder presses as long as you maintain your posture throughout the entire lift; focus on keeping the abs tight on the way up, and the back engaged on the way down. It's OK to lean backwards a little during the press—you'll need to for most styles of barbell shoulder press—but your upper body position should be relatively fixed during the movement. If you find yourself bending more backwards to lift the weight as the movement progresses, reduce the weight by a little bit so that you can lift the weight without needing to arch your back. Otherwise, you might risk losing your balance or injuring your back.

TRICEPS EXTENSION—With the elbows bent and holding the weight in your hands behind your head, extend your triceps (i.e., straighten your elbow), then return to the original position.

- Can be performed with a barbell, single dumbbell, or two dumbbells. Can be performed while standing, seated, or lying.
- Muscle group(s) worked: Triceps.
- Variation:
  - ♦ Triceps extension or pushdown machines.

- Pointers: squeeze your triceps for a full second at the end of the movement. When using machines, try bringing the weight back slowly, for a full 3-second count.

"HOW DO I GET RID OF SAGGY ARMS?"

Triceps workouts! Saggy arms are caused by a combination of loose skin and lack of muscle definition in the triceps area. Believe it or not, losing fat without adding muscle to this area will only make your arm skin more loose and saggy. Increasing the size of your triceps muscles will fill up the area, making the arm skin more taut.

UPRIGHT ROW—With the upper body completely vertical, hold weights with an overhand grip starting at the natural rest position below the waist and lift it straight up to the collarbone. Then return it to its original position.

- Can be performed with barbell or a dumbbell, while standing or seated, but is easiest to perform standing.
- Muscle group(s) worked: Shoulders. Shrugging your shoulders during the movement works out your traps (the lower neck muscles) too, so make sure you don't do this if you don't want the back of your neck getting more muscular. The muscles that are worked don't vary too much between standing or seated but be mindful not to swing your upper body to assist with the first half of the lift when standing.
- Pointers: As you drive your elbows upwards during the first half of this movement, it is important to keep your shoulders down; if you feel like you are shrugging as the weight comes up, you are working the wrong muscles. If you find that you can't bring the weights to your nipple line without shrugging your shoulders, lower the amount of weight until you can do so. To prevent swinging, hold the weight at the top of the movement for one second.

LOWER BODY

There are four main muscle groups that are emphasized during a leg workout. They are the gluteal muscles ("glutes" for short), the quadriceps ("quads" for short), the hamstrings, and the calves. Since the muscles that make up the buttock area consist of the gluteal muscles, we will refer to the glutes as the "butt" from here on out.

ABDUCTOR MACHINE—A seated workout machine that provides resistance as your push your legs apart at the hips.

- Muscle group(s) worked: Butt.
- Pointer: Squeeze your butt at the end of the movement and hold for one second. Bring your legs back to center slowly for a 3-second count.
- Variation:
  - *Seated Resistance Band Hip Abduction*—Sitting up tall in a chair, wrap a resistance band around the bottom of your thighs right above the top of your knees, with your knees hip width apart. Slowly push your knees out to the sides as you squeeze your butt. When you reach the end of the movement, continue to squeeze your butt and hold the movement for a second before bringing your legs back together, in a controlled motion.

HAMSTRING CURL/LEG CURL MACHINE—With the lower legs flexed against resistance, pull your heel to your butt.

- Muscle group(s) worked: Hamstrings.
- Pointer: Squeeze your butt at the top of the movement and hold for one second. Release the weight slowly for a 3-second count.

HIP THRUST—Start seated on the floor, knees bent, feet slightly wider than hip-distance apart. The upper back should be resting against the edge of a bench near its center (lengthwise). Lying on the floor with your knees bent and your feet flat on the ground, the hips are straightened in a thrusting motion to a fully extended position where the hips, shoulders, and knees are all in line before they return to their original positions.

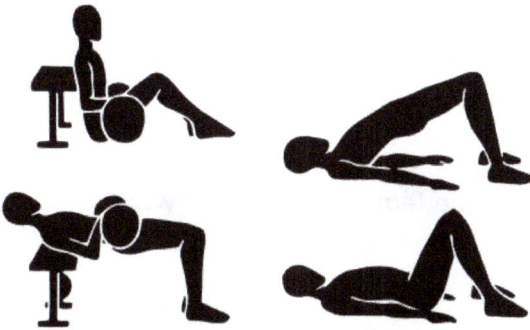

Figure 1 – Example of a Hip Thrust (left figures) vs. a Glute Bridge (right figures)

- Can be performed with a barbell or a dumbbell.
- Muscle groups worked: Butt.
- Variation:
  - *Glute Bridge*—The glute bridge is just like a hip thrust but performed without the bench and with your body on the ground. Lie down on your back with your knees bent and your feet flat on the ground, shoulder-width apart. Keeping your shoulders and feet planted on the floor, the hips are thrusted up and out until your body forms a straight line from your knees to your shoulders. Glute bridges tend to be more beginner friendly, but both exercises work

more or less the same muscles. You can get a bigger range of motion with hip thrusts, which is why it's my personal preference.

- Pointers: For both the glute bridge and hip thrust, squeeze your butt the entire time you are lifting your hips for maximum benefit. Keep your neck neutral as much as possible to avoid injury. Also, for both movements, raise your hips until your body forms a straight line from your knee to your hip and to your shoulder. Don't thrust beyond this point as this can reduce the effectiveness of the exercise.

LEG EXTENSION MACHINE—From a seated position with the legs bent, the legs are extended while under resistance before returning to the original position.

- Muscle group(s) worked: Quads.
- Pointer: Extend your leg almost completely at the end of the movement but do not lock them out. Hold at the top for one second. Release the weight slowly for a 3-second count.

LUNGE—Bring one leg forward and the other behind your body, keeping them hip-distance apart. Bend both knees, lowering your body toward the ground then return back to the starting position.

- Can be performed with barbell or a dumbbell
- Muscle group(s) worked: Butt, hamstrings, and quads with some attention to the calves.
- Variations:
  ♦ Walking
  ♦ In Place

- *Rear Foot Elevated/Bulgarian Split Squat*—Similar to the lunge in terms of muscles that are worked, but since your feet are static the whole move, you can focus on strength over balance and coordination. Raising the rear foot makes this movement more difficult than an in-place lunge because now you will need to engage your abs to stay balanced throughout the move. For an added challenge, try holding a single dumbbell during the movement. Regardless of which hand (planted side or non-planted side), you'll need to use your abs even more to stay balanced.
- *Front Foot Elevated*—gives you a deeper knee bend, putting more emphasis on the quad

- Pointers: Much like with a squat, make sure the knee of the planted foot tracks over your toes.

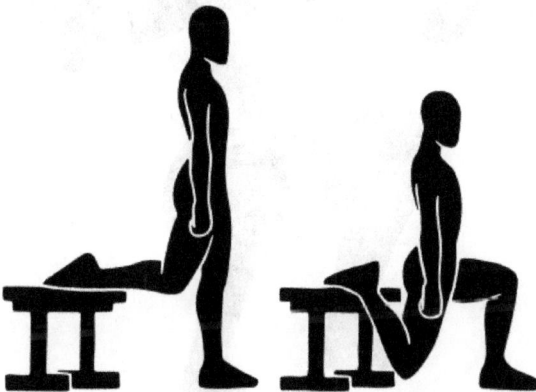

Figure 2 – Lunge Variation: the Rear Foot Elevated Lunge or Bulgarian Split Squat.

SQUAT—Stand with your feet just wider than hip-width apart, toes pointed slightly out. Keeping your upper body upright, lower your body by bending at the knees, as if to sit down. Then straighten your knees to return to the standing position.

- Can be performed with a barbell, a dumbbell, or kettlebell.
- Muscle group(s) worked: Mostly quads, hamstrings, and butt. Some abs and lower back
- Pointers: Given how important the squat is, there's a whole section below dedicated just to it.

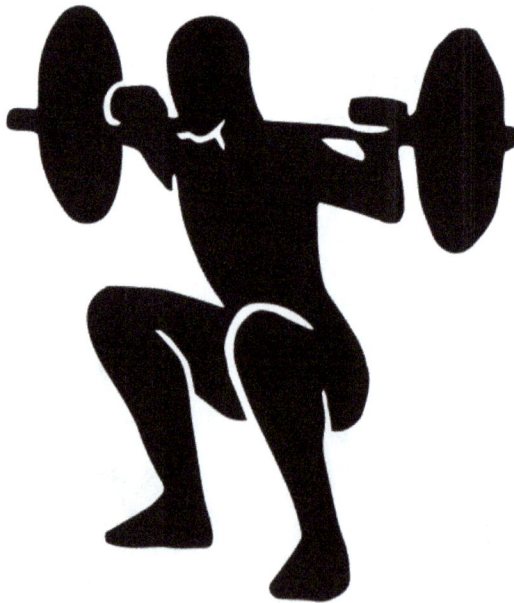

Figure 3 – An Example of Safe Squat Form: the thigh bone descends to a position that is slightly below parallel to the horizon and although the knee bends beyond the toes, it is aligned with the foot. The neck and back are in a neutral position as the squatter descends.

THE PROPER SQUAT FORM FOR A NICE BOOTY

Most people know what a squat is, but there's so much bad advice out there on proper squat technique I just wanted to highlight some tips that, from a biomechanical perspective, will give you the nicest booty while also minimizing damage to your joints.

1. Turn your toes out 15 to 30 degrees. This aligns the quads and brings them into the strongest position for squatting.

2. Place your feet between shoulder-width apart to 2 inches wider than that. In general, a slightly wider stance is better for building the butt, but only if you're both flexible enough (meaning your knees can track over your feet throughout the entire descent) and have strong enough hip muscles to maintain this position throughout the movement.

3. Contrary to popular belief, it is safe and actually beneficial to extend your knees past your toes as you squat...as long as the knees remain aligned with your feet during the movement.

4. Maintain a neutral neck and back position during your descent. A neutral neck position during the squat will typically have you looking at the floor a few feet ahead of you. Doing this during the descent will help maintain a neutral back position which, in turn, helps protect your lower back and maintain your squat's efficiency. Some people may arch their neck or back slightly as they ascend, or stand, from the squat. This is usually safe

provided that a neutral neck and back position were maintained during the descent.

5. The goal is to squat a little lower than a position where your thigh bone is parallel to the ground, which works out both the hamstrings and the butt, and not just the quads. If you can't break parallel, lower the weight until you can.

6. Control your descent. Do not bounce at the bottom! This is a common way that people injure their knees. This doesn't mean that you need to squat slowly; you just should not feel like you are falling or diving into the bottom of your squat.

7. Things to Avoid
   ♦ *Back rounding.* Rounding your back while squatting can not only lower your squat efficiency, but can also increase your chances of hurting your back. Rounding of the lower back, often called "butt wink," happens when one tucks their butt underneath their body at the bottom of the squat. This is often caused by immobility in ankle dorsiflexion (lack of ankle flexibility when pulling your foot closer to your shin) or poor hip mobility. Butt wink can often be improved by stretching your calves to improve your ankle mobility, widening your stance to reduce the amount of ankle flexibility required, or stretching your inner thighs to improve hip mobility. Rounding of the mid or upper back is typically indicative of a weak core during the lift. This can be improved by focusing on engaging your stomach and back muscles during the lift so that your upper body does not cave in or droop forward as you squat.

- *Knee caving/valgus collapse.* Make sure that your knees do not cave in as you descend into the squat as this can potentially lead to short- and long-term knee damage or knee pain. As you descend into the squat, your knee should track along with your foot as it bends; if you can see your toes on the *outside* of your knee as your knee bends, that is valgus collapse. Often, this is a sign that you are squatting with too heavy of a weight. Should you experience knee caving during the squat, lower the weight until you can squat without this happening. (Note: some knee caving as you ascend or stand up from the squat is safe for your knees, provided that (1) it does not cause you knee pain and (2) it is not so drastic that it causes you to table top your upper body during the movement.)

- *Bow-leggedness/varus knee.* While bow-leggedness is less common than knee caving when squatting, it also has the potential to cause short- and long-term knee damage or knee pain. If you can see your toes on the *inside* of your knee as your knees bend, that is a valgus knee position.

- *Folding forward or "table topping"* during the squat. A lot of lifters lean forward during the bottom of the descent because their hamstrings are not strong enough to support the weight. This is one of the most common errors for new lifters and a potential way to injure the lower back. Instead, engage your abs and lats to make sure that your upper body stays upright throughout the entire lift. If you find that you can't complete a squat without table topping, lower the weight to something that you can squat without doing so or strengthen your hamstrings with some hamstring curls.

- *Extreme neck positions*. Avoid looking straight down (doing this can lead to a pulled back) or looking straight up (this can reduce your technique efficacy) during the descent of the squat.

While we're here, are there other ways to better build a bodacious booty?

The muscles of your butt are designed to do two things: hinge your upper body back and forth (the muscles are needed for returning to upright) and opening (abducting) your legs at the hips. Therefore, the best exercises to build your butt include a hinge motion (try alternating between the Romanian deadlift and the squat) and an abduction motion (the abductor machine and seated hip abduction with a resistance band work the best for this).

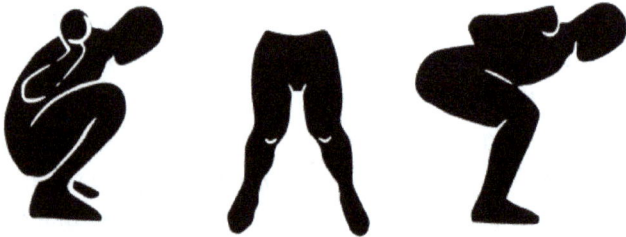

Figure 4 – 3 examples of Techniques to Avoid When Squatting (from left to right): 1. Lower back rounding/butt wink. 2. Knee caving/valgus collapse. 3. Forward folding/ table topping.

STEP-UPS—Step onto a raised platform with one foot, lifting your entire body as well as your back foot up onto the step. Then step backward to the starting position.

- Can be performed with bodyweight or while holding dumbbells.
- Muscles worked: Butt, hamstrings, and quads.
- Variation:
  - ♦ Single Leg Chair Squats.

- Pointers: The higher the step, the more challenging the exercise, so pick a step height that is challenging but safe for you. For me, a step that requires me to lift my knee to hip height is ideal. Regardless of the step height, to get the full benefit of this movement, step up using only your stepping foot instead of pushing off the back foot.

BACK

There are four major muscle groups that we tend to associate with back exercises. They are the trapezius, the rhomboids, the latissimus dorsi ("lat" or "lats" for short), and the erector spinae ("erectors" for short). For simplicity, we will refer to the trapezius and the rhomboids as the "upper back" and the lats as the "mid back" due to their relative locations on the body. While the erector spinae technically span your entire back along the spine, most of the erector exercises here will emphasize the lower erectors so for purposes of this book, we will refer to them as the "lower back."

BACK HYPEREXTENSIONS—With your feet anchored in the hyperextension bench, your upper body begins hinged forward, then extends to a straightened position.

- Muscle group(s) worked: lower back and some butt and hamstrings when the back is straight. Mostly the butt and some hamstrings when the upper back is relaxed.
- The back hyperextension can be performed with bodyweight or while holding a barbell, dumbbell, or kettlebell. To make it a butt-building exercise, emphasize squeezing your butt while keeping the upper body relaxed throughout the movement. Relaxing your upper back by slightly rounding your shoulders forward puts the focus of the exercise on the butt, while straightening the back puts the focus on your lower back. For both variations of this exercise, turning out the feet to 45 degrees increases the focus of the movement on the butt while reducing it on the hamstrings.

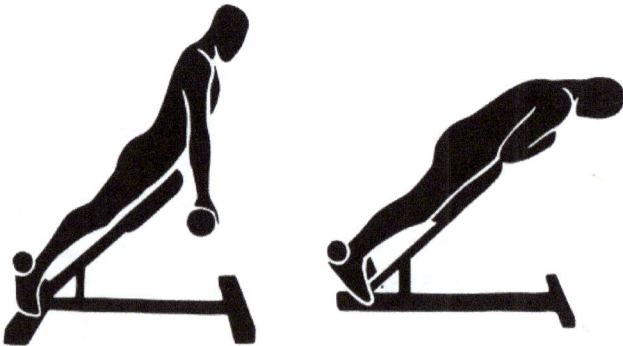

Figure 5 – Back Hyperextension Variations (from left to right):
1. Final position for the lower back focused variation
2. Final position for the butt focused variation. Feet may be rotated 45 degrees outward for more emphasis on butt building as shown in Variation 1.

PULL-UPS—While hanging from a bar with your body extended fully and your palms facing away from you, pull yourself up until your chin is above the bar.

- Muscle group(s) worked: Mostly upper back. Some biceps.
- Variations:
  - ◆ Lat Pulldown Machine.
  - ◆ Pulls-Ups With Resistance Band Assistance.

- Pointer: Squeeze your back and hold your position at the bottom of the movement for a full second.

HOW TO DO A PULL-UP: EXERCISE PROGRESSIONS

The exercises below will help you build the necessary strength and technique needed to eventually do pull-ups. You may do a combination of any or all of them, depending on what equipment you have available.

1. Lat pulldowns using a lat pulldown machine: 4 sets of 8 reps
   - ◆ Pointers: Squeeze your upper back and hold your position at the bottom of the movement for 1 second, then release slowly for a 3-second count

2. Pull-Up Machine with a 3-Second Controlled Eccentric: 4 sets of 8 reps
   - ◆ This is a reverse pull-up; instead of pulling yourself up to the bar, you start from the bar and lower yourself slowly.
   - ◆ Scientific evidence shows that the negative/release portion of the lift (the "eccentric" phase) builds more

muscle than the concentric portion (which would be the pulling portion of the pull-up) and that by lengthening the duration of the eccentric phase of each rep, we can further increase muscle growth. As you get stronger, you can increase the eccentric time to 5 seconds per rep. From there, the next progression would be to decrease the amount of assistance from the pull-up machine and restart with a 3 second eccentric.

3. Resistance Band Assisted Pull-Up: 4 sets of As Many Reps As Possible
   ♦ Secure a resistance band around a pull-up bar. Put your foot or knee into the band and pull yourself up. Squeeze your upper back for 1-second at the top and lower yourself slowly over a 3-second count.

SEATED ROW MACHINE—The lower body remains fixed as you sit on this machine and pull the weighted horizontal cable in a row motion.

- This is performed on a cable machine, using a V-grip attachment. When gripping the attachment, your hands should be in a neutral grip (palms facing each other), a little more than half a foot apart.
- Muscle group(s) worked: Mostly mid-back. Some biceps.
- Variation:
  ♦ *Dumbbell Chest Supported Row* using a neutral grip.

- Pointers: Keep your elbows against your body and your shoulders back and down during the pull. Avoid flaring your elbows out, which engages the biceps instead of the back. Maintain a neutral back and avoid swinging or leaning backwards during the pull; your upper body position, except for your arms, should remain static during the movement. At the end of the pull, hold the position and squeeze your back muscles for one second. Release the weight slowly for a 3-second count.

ABDOMINALS

HANGING LEG RAISE—Suspend and stretch your body with an overhand grip on a bar so that you are hanging straight. Keeping your legs together and stretched, raise them gradually to parallel the floor and lower them back in the same manner. You can make the movement easier by bending your knees as you lift your legs.

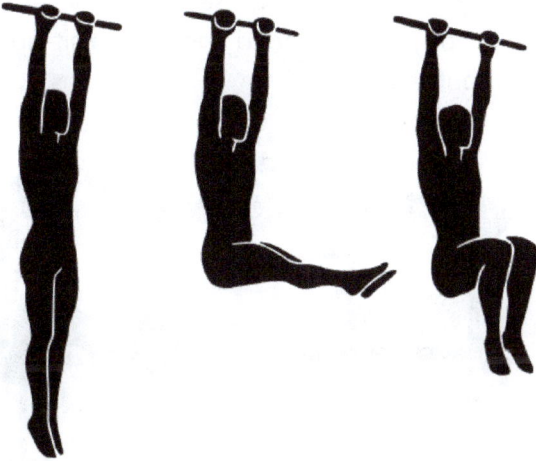

Figure 6 – Hanging Leg Raise (from left to right): 1. Starting position. 2. Final position with the legs stretched. 3. Final position of an easier variation with the knees bent.

- Muscle group(s) worked: Abs.
- Variations (hardest to easiest):

◆ *Lying Leg Raise*—A similar movement that is performed while lying face-up on the floor with your hands supporting your back. The legs are straight and lifted off the floor to the ceiling then returned to starting position.

◆ *Reverse Crunch*—Lying face-up on the floor with your arms by your sides and your knees bent at 90 degrees, raise your hips off the ground and pull your knees towards your chest while your upper body remains stationary against the floor. Knees are tucked toward your face as far as you can comfortably go without lifting your mid-back from the mat before they are slowly returned to their starting position.

HORIZONTAL HYPEREXTENSION SIT-UPS/HORIZONTAL ROMAN CHAIR SIT-UPS—This apparatus secures your legs in place so that your body is suspended and can do sit-ups without any back or butt support.

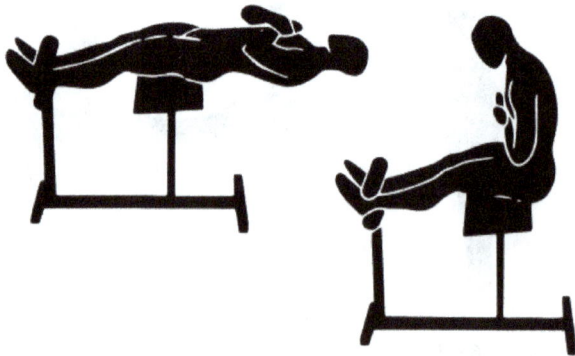

Figure 7 – Horizontal Hyperextension Sit-ups/Horizontal Roman Chair Sit-Ups

• Muscle group(s) worked: Abs.

- Variation:
  - ♦ *Decline Sit-Up*. These are a great alternative as you can adjust the decline position according to your strength level. The greater the bench is inclined, the harder it will be to perform the exercise, and vice versa.

- Pointers: For either exercise, make sure that you are not excessively rounding your upper or lower back during the movement. Slight rounding of the upper back is fine and safe, but the more you round your upper back, the more this becomes an upper ab exercise. Rounding of the lower back (which feels like tucking your butt in) increases the risk of injuring your lower back.

PLANK—A static hold in which you hold your body in a straight and in-line push-up-like position on your forearms, elbows, and toes.

- Muscle group(s) worked: Abs.
- Variation:
  - ♦ *Plank on Stability Ball*, with or without arm movement.

- Pointers: Don't let your hips sag as you perform this movement. Think about elongating your spine behind you as if you're pulling your tailbone towards your feet as a way to maintain your position.

HOW TO GET A SIX-PACK

When it comes to developing visible abs, especially for women, leanness matters more than muscle mass. Unfortunately, sit-ups alone won't get you a six-pack if you have too much abdominal fat.

In fact, building ab muscles will increase the size of your waist. Therefore, doing sit-ups without losing weight will produce the opposite result of a smaller waistline! Ab muscles won't be visible without achieving 10% (men) or 15% (women) leanness. If your goal is aesthetics, focus on building ab muscles only after you've hit the leanness threshold.

However, if you're at your desired leanness, you will just need 3 sets of one exercise per workout. Doing 8–12 reps per set three times a week will yield noticeable results. I find the fully horizontal Roman chair sit-up to be the most effective at building ab muscles, perhaps due to the difficult range of movements.

Planks on a stability ball also work well. For added difficulty, make slow and controlled circular movements on the stability ball with your arms while keeping the abs engaged.

WHOLE BODY

The deadlift is often hailed as the "King of All Lifts" since it's one of the few lifts that trains both upper and lower body muscles in one motion. However, for the exact same reasons that the deadlift is a great overall strength and muscle building exercise, it is also *difficult to perform correctly and prone to injury if done incorrectly.*

If you are reading this guide, you may be a beginner to strength training. For recreational lifters and those just looking to get in shape and not necessarily compete, *I recommend avoiding the deadlift unless you can learn proper technique with a qualified coach.* While it is indeed a powerful and versatile lift, it is *not* something to be trifled with.

Fortunately, two easier variations of the deadlift more suitable for beginners exist. In order of difficulty (harder to easier), these are the Stiff-Leg Deadlift ("SLDL") and the Romanian Deadlift ("RDL"). Both movements are less taxing versions of the conventional deadlift because they use fewer total muscle groups.

The SLDL and RDL are very similar movements in terms of body mechanics and muscles worked. The primary difference is that the RDL has a shorter range of movement and, for that reason, is easier for most beginners. The SLDL starts from the floor and the weight returns to a dead-stop position on the floor between each rep. Alternatively, during the RDL, the weight is lowered to just below the knees on each rep. At no point during the RDL does the weight touch the floor. The RDL is essentially the isolated hip-hinging portion of the deadlift exercise, the very portion of the lift from which the butt gets the biggest workout. While both deadlift variations do a great job working out your back, butt, and hamstrings, and the RDL is a particularly great beginner technique if you want to focus on building your butt.

STANDARD DEADLIFT—Weight is picked up off the ground to upper thigh level with your arms straight then returned to the floor.

- Can be performed with a barbell, dumbbells, or kettlebell
- Muscle group(s) worked: Lower, mid, and upper back. Butt, hamstrings, and quads.

STIFF-LEG DEADLIFT (SLDL)—Here, the quads are not used, with the primary focus being on the lower back and hamstrings, and the secondary focus on the butt. There is much less upper back engagement than in a conventional deadlift.

- Can be performed with a barbell, dumbbells, or kettlebell.
- Muscle group(s) worked: Mostly lower back, butt, and hamstrings. Some mid and upper back.

ROMANIAN DEADLIFT (RDL)—Again, the quads are not used; instead, the primary focus is on the butt, with the secondary focus being the lower back and hamstrings. There is much less upper back engagement than in a conventional deadlift.

- Can be performed with a barbell, dumbbells, or kettlebell.
- Muscle group(s) worked: lower back, butt, and hamstrings. Some mid and upper back.

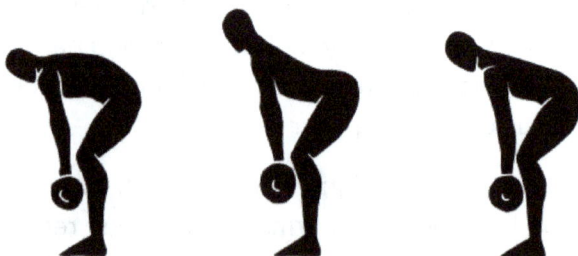

Figure 8 - The Deadlift (from left to right): excessive rounding of the back, excessive arching of the back, and the ideal neutral back position.

POINTERS FOR THE DEADLIFT AND ITS VARIATIONS

- These lifts can all be performed with a barbell, a kettlebell, or two dumbbells (one in each hand). For dumbbells, hold the dumbbells in front of the shin to mimic the placement of a barbell rather than out to the sides of your body.

- Stand with your feet hip-width apart. Bend your knees slightly, and then keep them rigid (do not change the angle of the bend) for the duration of your set.

- Push your butt back as you hinge your upper body forward from your hips in a controlled and slow manner, lowering the weight down past your knees towards the floor as far as your flexibility allows. You will feel your weight shift backwards slightly towards your heel, but your entire foot should still remain planted on the ground; if your toes come up off the floor as you hinge, you are overdoing it.

- When lowering the weight, keep it close to your legs by lowering it straight downward. The weight should not move away from the body (this indicates that your back is not engaged during the descent) nor does it need to graze your thighs (this could lead to excessive arching of the back).

- Do not round or arch your back during this movement as doing either increases your chance of pulling your lower back. Your back should remain neutral as you hinge forward. Keep your head neutral (look at the floor a few feet ahead of you) during the movement as well to prevent rounding or arching of the back. If you feel your upper back rounding during the entire descent, then you've picked a weight that is too heavy for your back. If you feel your lower back rounding towards the bottom of your hinge position, then you've exceeded the limitations of your hip hinge (i.e., your hamstring flexibility). Once this happens, the tension moves from the butt and hamstrings to your lower back; this is not always a bad thing, but it may put you at more risk of harming your lower back if you are not careful. Stop your descent right before you reach this point.

- Squeeze your butt as you drive your hips forward and stand up.

THE WORKOUT PLANS

For all workouts listed, each workout should take less than an hour including the warmups.

BOLDED EXERCISES are the most taxing on your body. Don't skip these; they are the biggest return on investment for your work, both from a calorie burning and muscle building perspective.

- You should do one or two sets of warm-up sets at a lower weight for these exercises, so expect them to take up the biggest amount of time in your workout.
- These exercises should be done first, and the other exercises may be performed in whatever order you'd like.
- If you are in a hurry and can't complete the entire workout, perform the exercise in bold for the biggest bang for your buck and skip one of the unbolded exercises; just don't skip the same exercise every time or you risk underdeveloped muscle groups and asymmetry.

- If you plan to do intense cardio, do it *after* lifting, so you aren't too tired to lift.

2-DAY BEGINNER WORKOUT

Good for people going to the gym for the first time or getting back to working out after a long hiatus.

- Back and Lower Body Day:
  - ♦ **Squats**, 4 sets of 8–10 reps
  - ♦ Back hyperextensions (either variation), 4 sets of 10–12 reps
  - ♦ Lat pulldowns, 4 sets of 10–12 reps
  - ♦ Dumbbell lunges, 4 sets of 10–12 reps per leg

- Upper Body Day:
  - ♦ **Pick one: barbell or dumbbell** bench presses, incline benches, Arnold presses, or shoulder presses, **4 sets of 8–10 reps**
  - ♦ Upright rows, 4 set of 10 reps
  - ♦ One biceps exercise (such as curls), 4 sets of 10 reps
  - ♦ One triceps exercise (such as triceps extensions), 4 set of 10 reps

3-DAY WHOLE BODY WORKOUT

Solid workout for anyone. Each workout takes about an hour.

- Leg day:
  - ♦ **Squats**, 4 sets of 8–10 reps
  - ♦ Dumbbell lunges, 4 sets of 10–12 reps each leg
  - ♦ Pick one: leg extensions or step-ups, 4 sets of 10 reps

- Pick one: hamstring curls, hip thrusts, or glute bridges, 4 sets of 10 reps

- Upper Body Day:
  - **Pick one: barbell or dumbbell** bench presses, incline benches, Arnold presses, or shoulder presses, 4 sets of 8–10 reps
  - Lateral raises, 3 sets of 10 reps
  - Rear delt flies, 3 sets of 10 reps
  - One biceps exercise (such as curls), 4 sets of 10 reps
  - One triceps exercise (such as triceps extensions), 4 set of 10 reps

- Core (Back and Abs) Day:
  - Pick one (in order from hardest to easiest): **stiff leg deadlifts** or back hyperextensions with engaged upper lats, 4 sets of 10 reps
  - Pick one (in order from hardest to easiest): assisted pull-ups, pull-up machine with 3-second descent, or lat pull-downs, 4 sets of 10 reps
  - Seated cable rows, 3 sets of 10 reps
  - For the lower abs, pick one (in order from hardest to easiest): horizontal Roman chair, hanging leg raises, leg lifts, reverse crunches, 3 sets of 10–12 reps
  - For upper abs: planks on a stability ball. Advanced version: make slow and controlled circular motions with your arms as you balance your body on the ball, 3 rounds of 30 seconds.

4-DAY WORKOUT

This workout is for those who have more time to commit. It takes the upper body day from the 3-day workout and splits it into two shorter workouts, with the second workout done after the back day:

- Upper Body Day 1:
  - ◆ Barbell or dumbbell bench presses, 3 sets of 8 reps
  - ◆ Barbell or dumbbell incline bench presses, 3 sets of 10 reps
  - ◆ One bicep exercise (such as curls), 3 sets of 10 reps
  - ◆ One triceps exercise (machine option: triceps push downs; dumbbell option: triceps extension with single dumbbell; bodyweight option: push-ups), 3 sets of 10 reps
  - ◆ One abdominal exercise, 3 sets of 10 reps

- Leg Day:
  - ◆ **Squats**, 4 sets of 8–10 reps
  - ◆ Dumbbell lunges, 4 sets of 10–12 reps each leg
  - ◆ Pick one: leg extensions or step-ups, 4 sets of 10 reps
  - ◆ Pick one: hamstring curls, hip thrusts, or glute bridges, 4 sets of 10 reps

- Upper Body Day 2:
  - ◆ Pick one (in order from hardest to easiest): barbell or dumbbell Arnold presses or shoulder presses, 3 sets of 8 reps
  - ◆ Barbell or dumbbell standing upright rows, 3 sets of 10 reps
  - ◆ Lateral raises, 3 sets of 10 reps
  - ◆ Rear delt flies, 3 sets of 10 reps

- One abdominal exercise: 3 sets of 10 reps

- Core (Back and Abs) Day:
  - Pick one (in order from hardest to easiest): **stiff leg deadlifts** or back hyperextensions with engaged upper lats, 4 sets of 10 reps
  - Pick one (in order from hardest to easiest): assisted pull-ups, pull-up machine with 3-second descent, or lat pull-downs, 4 sets of 10 reps
  - Seated cable rows, 3 sets of 10 reps
  - For the lower abs, pick one (in order from hardest to easiest): horizontal Roman chair, hanging leg raises, leg lifts, reverse crunches, 3 sets of 10–12 reps
  - For upper abs: planks on a stability ball. Advanced version: make slow and controlled circular motions with your arms as you balance your body on the ball, 3 rounds of 30 seconds.

To be worked in throughout the workout week:
  - 1 hour total intense cardio or 90 minutes of moderate cardio

3-DAY BIKINI BODY WORKOUT

This swimsuit-ready workout is focused on women who want to achieve a toned look.

- Leg Day:
  - **Squats**, 4 sets of 8–10 reps
  - Lunges, 3 sets of 10–12 reps for each leg
  - Abduction machine, 4 sets of 10–12 reps
  - Glute bridges or hip thrusts, 3 sets of 10 reps
  - Step-ups, 2 sets of 10 reps for each leg

- Upper Body Day:
  - ♦ Seated Dumbbell Shoulder presses, 3 sets of 12 reps
  - ♦ Upright rows, 3 sets of 10 reps
  - ♦ One biceps exercise (such as curls), 3 sets of 10 reps
  - ♦ One triceps exercise (machine option: triceps push downs, dumbbell option: I triceps extension with single dumbbell, bodyweight option: push-ups), 3 sets of 10 reps

- Core (Back and Abs) Day:
  - ♦ Pick one (in order from hardest to easiest): Romanian Deadlift or back hyperextension, 4 sets of 10 reps
  - ♦ Lat pull-downs or pull-up progression, 4 sets of 10–12 reps
  - ♦ For the lower abs, pick one (from hardest to easiest): horizontal Roman chair, hanging leg raises, leg lifts, reverse crunches, 3 sets of 10–12 reps
  - ♦ For upper abs: Planks on a stability ball. Advanced version: Make slow and controlled circular motions with your arms as you balance your body on the ball, 3 rounds of 30 seconds.

BODYWEIGHT WORKOUT

Working out when you have to travel, or have no access to equipment but want to get going:

- Push-ups, 3 sets to failure with 2-minute rest between each round
- Pick one, bodyweight squats or (advanced) jumping squats, 3 sets of 20 reps
- Walking lunges, 3 sets of 20 reps each side
- Step-ups onto a stool, 3 sets of 10 reps on each side

"THIS IS ALL STILL TOO HARD! HOW DO I FIND HELP?"

Don't feel bad about wanting to hire help! I've been lifting for over a decade and I've had a coach or a personal trainer the entire time. At first, it was because I didn't know how to train on my own and I was afraid of injuring myself. After a few years, it would be reasonable to think that I knew how to lift on my own, but quite frankly, I was too lazy to. At heart, I'm a very lazy person in the body of a person that doesn't want to be lazy (and that loves to spend money on trainers, apparently).

Most days, I know that if I don't pay a coach to train me, I either won't work out, or I'll do a half-assed job of it. So for me, at first the money initially spent was worth it to learn how to exercise safely. Now it's worth it because I'm buying the discipline that I intrinsically don't have.

For the same reasons—learning to exercise safely and keeping to your goals—you might want to consider hiring a trainer. As previously indicated, I know that hiring fitness support can be expensive. Below are some ways to try to make it work. Consider trying a variety of options as your time and resources allow:

- Try remote coaching instead of in-person coaching.

- Pay for short-term personal training just to learn proper form and technique for specific exercises. To make the best use of your time and money, predetermine which exercises you want to learn with your coach before committing to sessions.

- Attend one or two-day fitness seminars.

- Attend group barbell or weightlifting classes at CrossFit or strength training gyms.

How to pick the right trainer:

- Don't just go by how they look. Some people naturally have great physiques without needing to do much.

- Ask about their athletic history and resume. Ideally, the person you currently work with is or once was an athlete themselves, and has actual bodybuilding or powerlifting experience.

- Look at their clients. Ask if you can see or meet some of their current clients, not just their best success stories. If these coaches are at all competent at what they claim, they should have a variety of clients who are:

  ♦ Bodybuilders, powerlifters, or athletes who perform compound lifts like football players; this is the bare minimum proof (but not a guarantee) that they know how to teach lifting technique.

  ♦ Healthy and injury free.

  ♦ Better looking after than they were before they started training.

- A competent coach will also have long term client retention; if clients are leaving every six months, they are either getting injured or just not seeing positive results.

Most importantly, the best coach will be responsive and have enough bandwidth to help you. Neophyte lifters will need the most handholding when it comes to learning proper technique, so you want a coach who will be reasonably available to provide real-time feedback to help you not injure yourself. Unfortunately, some of the most well-known coaches in the industry are overwhelmed and, as a result, do not respond in a timely or thoughtful way to their clients. At best you'll get a few minutes of their time every week, and they won't give much attention to detail in critiquing your form. This can be frustrating, unmotivating, dangerous, and a poor use of your time and money.

A LESS COSTLY ALTERNATIVE FOR FEEDBACK ON YOUR FORM

Hiring a personal trainer can be a prohibitively expensive way of getting feedback on your form. As an alternative, there are virtual options in which you can film yourself performing a technique and then send it to a coach for feedback—at a fraction of the cost. This is a worthwhile investment for a beginner as there's nothing more unmotivating to getting in shape than hurting yourself in the process.

PART 3

SLEEP

Sleep is the most underrated of all dietary tools. And yet, while it's something that we all do, not everyone is naturally good at it.

Sleep is easily the most powerful and perhaps easiest way to improve the effectiveness of your diet and your workouts. Most adults need 7 to 9 hours of sleep a night to not feel sleep-deprived. However, getting sufficient sleep is not just about sleeping enough hours, it's also about getting good quality sleep.

How Sleep Deprivation Keeps You From the Results You Want

For the sake of simplicity, we will define sleep deprivation here as "insufficient sleep, lack of sleep, sleep loss, poor sleep quality, or short sleep duration."

Most of us already know firsthand that sleep deprivation can negatively affect our moods. But beyond ruining our day, poor sleep can also ruin our long-term health. Indeed, chronic sleep deprivation of as little as one hour per night has been linked to an increase in hypertension, diabetes, obesity, depression, heart attack, stroke, and all-cause mortality. With respect to diet and fitness, sleep deprivation negatively impacts many hormones, including the hormones involved with appetite, stress, metabolism, fertility, and muscle repair and building. It has also been found to trigger increased levels of the hormone ghrelin, which controls your hunger, leading to increased appetite.

Sleep deprivation has also been found to have negative impacts on your brain functions, including critical thinking, logic, decision making, and impulse control. On one level, dieting is all about controlling the impulse to eat what we want to eat over what we logically should eat. Separate scientific studies have shown that adults who on average increase the number of hours they sleep each night have an easier time reducing their calorie intake, and that those who are sleep-deprived tend to consume more overall calories. Put simply, a lack of sleep combined with increased hunger makes you more likely to overeat and make poor nutritional choices.

Another way sleep deprivation hurts our physique goals is by reducing the hormones that stimulate muscle growth and repair, thereby potentially also reducing muscle mass and strength. Not good—not good for the diet, not good for the workout.

This is all just a long-winded way of saying that if you ever have to pick between a full night of sleeping and getting a workout in, pick the extra sleep! It'll be more beneficial to your health, diet, and strength in the long run.

Scientifically validated and recommended ways to improve your sleep include:

- Go to bed at the same time every night and wake up at the same time in the morning. The body's internal processes follow a 24-hour clock called the circadian rhythm that regulates the sleep-wake cycle and all the bodily functions in between. The circadian rhythm relies heavily on consistency. A consistent bedtime will help train your body's internal clock to know around what time it should start feeling sleepy every night. This will also help you get enough time in each of the four stages of sleep (falling asleep, light sleep, slow wave sleep/deep sleep, and REM sleep), which is necessary for optimal health.

- Use your bed only for sleeping. This is more for Pavlovian training than it is your circadian rhythm. Many people like to eat, watch TV, read, and lounge in bed. However, if you only enter your bed when you are about to sleep, this will condition your body into associating your bed with sleepy feelings. It may sound a little silly, but your mind is very powerful when it comes to building habits. As best as you can, remove all non-sleeping activities (except for sex, of course) from your bed.

- Take magnesium before bed for better sleep. I like magnesium L-threonate (a more stable and bioavailable form of magnesium, speculated to be better for brain health) or magnesium glycinate for sleep, as they are both easily absorbed and have no laxative effect. Other forms, like magnesium malate, can have a laxative effect.

- Don't eat a heavy or fatty meal within 2 hours of sleeping. After a big meal, your body needs several hours to digest food, which otherwise will slow down the start of the sleep process and actually decrease that evening's sleep quality and amount. It also increases the possibility of sleep disruptions and acid reflux. If you're feeling hungry before you sleep, eat something slow-digesting yet light, like a protein shake, a slice of high fiber toast, or some almonds.

- Stop caffeine at lunchtime. Caffeine has a long half-life of 5 to 6 hours, so it takes a long time for all of it to leave your body. If you drink coffee at 4 p.m., you may still be stimulated at 10 p.m.!

- Exercising can have a stimulating effect, so stop exercising 3 hours before bedtime to keep your body relaxed and your core body temperature low when you hit the sack.

- Try to relax instead of electronically stimulating your eyes and nervous system in the hour leading up to bed. Avoid handheld electronic devices, and reduce all screen time including your TV, smartphone, and computer. (It is thought that blue light from electronic devices is particularly bad for sleep.) Try other activities in the hour before bed, like meditation or journaling. Trying to get work done or entertaining yourself through screens will make it harder to sleep.

- Avoid alcohol consumption. Many people think that a drink or two at night helps them sleep better. This is not completely true: while it is true that alcohol can help you fall asleep, even a small amount of alcohol before going to bed will reduce your sleep quality and the duration of your sleep. A very large sleep study of over 4,000 adults found that two servings of alcohol per day for men or one serving per day for women decreased sleep quality by 24%. Additionally, many scientific studies have also observed that alcohol consumption reduces your rapid eye movement (REM) sleep for that evening, which is the phase of sleep that stimulates the areas of your brain that are essential for learning and making or retaining memories. In short, any benefit that alcohol may provide in helping you fall asleep is greatly outweighed by its negative effect on sleep quality.

- If you wake up in the middle of the night, it's better to get out of bed then stay in it with your mind running and body tossing and turning. Find a chair or couch and sit for a little while, and then when you get tired again, come back to bed. In this way, your subconscious mind won't come to associate bed with being a place where your mind runs and your body tosses and turns.

If you find implementing this whole list to be somewhat difficult, feel free to pick and choose the sleep pointers that you can work into your daily routine. Admittedly, on any given day, I sometimes don't adhere to all of the guidelines, even more so when I'm traveling. But I do notice that the more regularly I follow most of the guidelines, the better my overall quality of sleep.

PART 4

SUPPLEMENTS

Some people treat supplements like magic pills and expect to fix whatever problems they have by popping a few of them into their mouth. However, the name "supplements" itself is a direct pointer: they are meant to *supplement* your activities and your body's needs.

What supplements do we actually need when working out, and how do they help? The following recommendations are backed by scientific research and have been found to be safe within the recommended doses. I also list the potential side effects for each substance.

PRE-WORKOUT SUPPLEMENTS

While pre-workout supplements are definitely not necessary to have a good workout, I do enjoy the physical and mental boosts that they can provide. I take all of the following 20 to 30 minutes before I work out. The list may look very long and intimidating, but the first four compounds are commonly found together in many pre-workout powders:

- **CAFFEINE**—A compound found in plants that works as a stimulant for the nervous system

PROS: Caffeine increases your power output, exercise performance, pain tolerance, endurance, and can help you feel more alert and enhance your focus.

CONS: *Caffeine's half-life is up to 5 hours.* If you take it too late in the day, it will negatively affect your sleep.

Recommended dosage: 100–200 mg (equivalent to a medium coffee shop coffee or two home brewed cups of coffee).

- **CREATINE**—A compound found in living tissues that keeps a constant supply of energy to the muscles.

PROS: Creatine is one of the most well-researched and effective workout supplements. A very large number of scientific studies show that it increases explosive power with no negative side effects.

CONS: Creatine increases water retention in the muscles so *it may make your muscles look bigger and buffer.* Many men seem to enjoy this side effect, but for those who aren't going for the "swole" look, you may want to avoid this supplement.

Recommended dosage: 3–5 g a day, depending on your weight.

- **BETA ALANINE**—An amino acid found in meat and made by the human body and a potential antioxidant.

PROS: It reduces the lactic acid (the compound your body produces during exercise that is associated with muscle fatigue) built up in your muscles during exercise. Several scientific studies also suggest it increases endurance.

CONS: Some people experience *tingling, itching, or blood vessel pumps* in their skin that feel uncomfortable. While these side effects are harmless and go away after a few hours, they can be undesirable and distracting if they happen during your workout!

Recommended dosage: 2–5 g a day.

"What are antioxidants and why are they so important?"

Antioxidants are chemicals that neutralize molecules in our body that can otherwise damage our cells. Without antioxidants, these molecules can damage our DNA and cause long-term health problems such as diabetes, heart disease, cancer, and neurodegenerative disease.

Common antioxidants that we can obtain through our diet include many of the daily vitamins and minerals recommended by the U.S. Food and Nutrition Board such as vitamin C, vitamin E, beta-carotene, selenium, and manganese.

- **L-CITRULLINE**—L-Citrulline is an amino acid found in food like watermelon and made by the human body. Citrulline malate, an organic salt of citrulline, is the same for our purposes, so we will refer to both products interchangeably as "citrulline" from here on out. Both of these forms of citrulline boost nitric oxide production in the body. The body converts citrulline to L-arginine, another type of amino acid. L-arginine (or arginine for short) improves blood flow by creating nitric oxide (NO), a gas that helps your arteries relax, thereby slightly lowering your blood pressure and increasing your blood flow. The extra blood flow is helpful because muscles that are being exercised require more blood to make the energy needed to power continuous muscle contractions.

PROS: Many scientific studies that suggest that the improved blood flow from citrulline results in increased power output, higher training volume, and decreased fatigue and soreness.

CONS: There are currently no known side effects for either form of citrulline when taken by healthy individuals.

Recommended dosage: 2–5 g a day for L-Citrulline, 3–8 g a day for citrulline malate.

"If I'm trying to increase my arginine levels, why don't I just take arginine?"

Due to our body's digestive track, oral citrulline is more bioavailable than oral arginine, so of the two supplements, citrulline is the more efficient way to increase blood flow. However, you can enhance the effects of either supplement by taking citrulline and arginine *together*: oral citrulline increases the bioavailability of arginine and rapidly raises arginine levels in the blood. Studies have shown that the combination of oral citrulline and arginine supplementation increased blood arginine more effectively than either supplement alone, leading to a significantly greater increase in nitric oxide in the blood, which also results in significantly increased blood flow.

Recommended arginine dosage when taking with citrulline: 2–4 g a day.

- **COLLAGEN TYPE 2**—Collagen type 2 is what cartilage is made of, while collagen types 1 and 3 serve as the building blocks of hair, skin, nails, tendons, ligaments, and bones.

  PROS: Studies show that taking collagen before a workout can temporarily reduce exercise-related joint pain (although it cannot rebuild cartilage). I take a powder blend of all three types every day before I work out to keep my joints feeling good and my skin and hair looking nice. Another added benefit of collagen powder is that it contains some protein, so I'll often add collagen to my morning coffee so that the protein in the collagen and in the milk in my coffee hold me over until lunch.

  CONS: Collagen powder is low-calorie but not calorie-free, so don't go crazy with it. Some people experience stomach aches with excess amounts. However, there is no unsafe dosage if that's a concern.

  Recommended dosage: 10 g a day.

  > TIP: Collagen is synthesized with vitamin C so for maximum benefit make sure you get enough vitamin C in your diet or you can take a supplement!

POST-WORKOUT SUPPLEMENTS

Rehydrating and restoring your energy levels are the only time-sensitive activities to worry about post-workout. When you sweat during a workout, your body loses both water and electrolytes (salts), most of which are sodium. The more strenuous your workout, the more of your body's sugar supplies get depleted as well. For this reason, most post-workout drinks are usually water with some added salt and sugar—not only are you putting back in what's lost, but both salt and sugar help your body retain water better than drinking water alone. This is also why people lose weight very quickly during the first week of a low-salt or low-carb diet: they are losing water weight and not actually losing fat.

You can opt for a sports drink or water to stay hydrated during your workout; either is fine as long as you feel hydrated enough. However, if you find yourself feeling very dehydrated during or after your workout, I would suggest that you consume a sports drink that has salt or electrolytes in it like sugar-free or regular Gatorade. If you find yourself incredibly winded during or after your workout, I would make sure to have a sports drink that has both salt and sugar in it, like regular Gatorade. For really strenuous workouts, eating a high carb meal immediately after working out might also help you recover your energy levels. (You may recall in Part 1 that I advise not to remove the carbs from your post-workout meal. This is why.)

NON-WORKOUT SUPPLEMENTS

I like the following supplements for maintaining good health, as they provide great general health benefits that are not necessarily exercise-specific:

- **CURCUMIN WITH BIOPERINE**—Curcumin is a natural compound that helps fight inflammation in our body and is the active ingredient found in the spice turmeric. Bioperine is a black pepper extract that significantly increases curcumin's absorption into the body. But before you ask, "Can I just add turmeric spice to all my foods instead?" let me clarify that turmeric spice in only about 3% curcumin, so unless you *really* like turmeric flavor in your food, I would recommend that you primarily get your curcumin from supplements and secondarily through spice.

PROS: This compound reduces inflammation and joint pain by increasing the body's ability to naturally make antioxidants.

CONS: This is a spice, so in general, no downsides as long as you aren't allergic to turmeric.

Recommended dosage: 1,000 mg a day.

- **FISH OIL**—A dietary source of omega-3 fatty acids eicosapentaenoic acid (EPA) and docosahexaenoic acid (DHA).

  PROS: Whether you work out or not, this supplement is good for you in general; strong scientific evidence has found that fish oil increases good cholesterol, lowers blood pressure, reduces depression, and lowers triglycerides (the fat in your blood that increases the risk of heart disease).

  CONS: While a good fat, it is still fat. And eating too much at once can give you bloat and gas!

  Recommended dosage: Pick a type with at least 1,000 mg EPA (a type of omega-3 fatty acid).

- **VITAMIN C**—Vitamin C is a water-soluble vitamin found in citrus fruits.

  PROS: This vitamin is used to prevent illnesses and is a powerful antioxidant.

  CONS: Some people experience digestive issues if they take too much (over 2,000 mg) of Vitamin C in one sitting. Don't worry, you'd have to consume 25 oranges to get to that level!

  Recommended dosage: 75 mg for women and 90 mg for men a day, which you can get and then some by eating two oranges or one bell pepper of any color. I'd recommend just eating a fruit or veggie high in vitamin C rather than taking a supplement, as plants high in vitamin C tend to have a lot of other healthy nutrients as well.

  > TIP: Take fish oil and curcumin supplements with food since these supplements are fat-soluble (absorption increases when paired with dietary fats). I take both supplements after lunch, but you can pick whichever meal is most convenient for you.

PART 5

"EFFORT, NOT PERFECTION"

Okay, so you've made it to the end of the book. Congratulations!

By now, you've absorbed a lot of information and I'm guessing it may seem pretty overwhelming. Sometimes, when I offer this kind of advice to my friends, they'll ask, "What if I can't do it all?" If you can't do everything every time, that's OK. Just do as much as you can given your current circumstances. You're not always going to be able to complete every task perfectly; life happens. If you fixate on perfection, the process of getting in better shape is going to be miserable and you're not going to stick with it.

It's understandable if some days this kind of advice feels unpleasant; there are days when even I don't want to work out. And there are even more days when I don't want to stick to my diet. On these days, I just do what I can. Typically, I'll either pick the easiest thing I can accomplish (just sleeping well) or the most important thing I need to accomplish for my current goal (getting in a good workout if I'm training for a competition). Even accomplishing just one of these tasks usually leaves me feeling good about myself for having done something that was, in fact, good for me.

Lifting is a huge stress reliever for me and I enjoy lifting more than I care about losing weight, so I would rather squeeze in time at the gym. However, if your main goal is to lose weight, I'd make getting enough sleep and following the diet as often as possible your main priority. Extra physical activity is great too, but if you can't make time for exercise, taking some extra footsteps every day still makes a difference.

FINAL THOUGHTS

In bringing together a decade's worth of health and fitness experience into one short book, I've summarized and presented the information in what I thought would be the easiest way for a fitness newcomer to understand. Of course, even advice that is easy to understand may not be easy to implement. It's not that most people don't have the time, resources, or even the will to get in shape; instead, all too often, something simply gets in the way and makes fitness hard. Nobody wants to have to pick between sticking with their diet and enjoying an event with friends or family. I certainly don't.

If anything, I hope the one thing that sticks with you from this book is that healthy living involves a spectrum of effort and is not defined by a single all-or-nothing event. Some days, you'll be able to follow your diet and fitness routine 100%, other days it will be 25%, but, hopefully, most days it can be at least 80%. As long as you know which efforts count the most towards achieving your goals—and which ones you can pragmatically fit into your daily life—you'll be able to find ways to create healthier daily habits that eventually make fitness feel more like an automatic experience, and less like an effort or an inconvenience.

And while health and fitness may never become completely automatic or easy for most of us, I hope that through the process of reading this book, it at least now feels a little easier and more possible for you.

Good luck on your fitness journey. You can do it!

REFERENCES

Agarwal, U., Didelija, I. C., Yuan, Y., Wang, X., & Marini, J. C. (2017). Supplemental Citrulline Is More Efficient Than Arginine in Increasing Systemic Arginine Availability in Mice. *The Journal of nutrition*, *147*(4), 596–602. https://doi.org/10.3945/jn.116.240382

American Heart Association. (2017, March 23). *Trans Fats*. American Heart Association. Retrieved August 23, 2022, from https://www.heart.org/en/healthy-living/healthy-eating/eat-smart/fats/trans-fat

Carbone, J. W., & Pasiakos, S. M. (2019). *Dietary Protein and Muscle Mass: Translating Science to Application and Health Benefit*. MDPI. Retrieved August 23, 2022, from https://doi.org/10.3390/nu11051136

Cheng, I. S., Wang, Y. W., Chen, I. F., Hsu, G. S., Hsueh, C. F., & Chang, C. K. (2016). The Supplementation of Branched-Chain Amino Acids, Arginine, and Citrulline Improves Endurance Exercise Performance in Two Consecutive Days. *Journal of sports science & medicine*, *15*(3), 509–515.

Ciuris, C., Lynch, H., Wharton, C., & Johnston, C. (2019). A Comparison of Dietary Protein Digestibility, Based on DIAAS Scoring, in Vegetarian and Non-Vegetarian Athletes.

Nutrients. 10.3390/nu11123016. PMID: 31835510; PMCID: PMC6950041.

Cognitive Vitality. (2016, Aug 31). *Magnesium Cognitive Vitality for Researchers.* Retrieved August 23, 2022, from https://www.alzdiscovery.org/uploads/cognitive_vitality_media/Magnesium-Cognitive-Vitality-For-Researchers.pdf

Ebrahim, I. O., Shapiro, C. M., Williams, A. J., & Fenwick, P. B. (2013). Alcohol and sleep I: effects on normal sleep. *Alcoholism, clinical and experimental research, 37*(4), 539–549. https://doi.org/10.1111/acer.12006

Examine. *Supplements.* Retrieved August 23, 2022, https://examine.com/supplements/

Ferrie, J. E., Shipley, M. J., Akbaraly, T. N., Marmot, M. G., Kivimäki, M., & Singh-Manoux, A. (2011). Change in sleep duration and cognitive function: findings from the Whitehall II Study. *Sleep, 34*(5), 565–573. https://doi.org/10.1093/sleep/34.5.565

Houdek, A. (2011, July 27). *The Paleo Diet: Caveman Cure-All or Unhealthy Fad?* The Atlantic. Retrieved August 23, 2022, from https://www.theatlantic.com/health/archive/2011/07/the-paleo-diet-caveman-cure-all-or-unhealthy-fad/242621/

House, J. D., Neufeld, J., & Leson, G. (2010). Evaluating the Quality of Protein from Hemp Seed (Cannabis sativa L.) Products Through the use of the Protein Digestibility-Corrected Amino Acid Score Method. *Journal of Agricultural and Food Chemistry, 58*(22), 11801-11807. 10.1021/jf102636b

Institute of Medicine (US) Committee on Sleep Medicine and Research; Colten HR, Altevogt BM, editors. Sleep Disorders and Sleep Deprivation: An Unmet Public Health Problem.

Washington (DC): National Academies Press (US); 2006. Available from: https://www.ncbi.nlm.nih.gov/books/ NBK19960/ doi: 10.17226/11617

Jäger, R., Kersick, C., Campbell, B., Wells, S., Skwiat, T., Purpura, M., Ziegenfuss, T., Ferrando, A., Arent, S., Smith-Ryan, A., Stout, J., Arciero, P., Ormsbee, M., Taylor, L., Wilborn, C., Kalman, D., Kreider, R., Willoughby, D., Hoffman, J., ... J Antonio. (2017, Jun 20). International Society of Sports Nutrition Position Stand: protein and exercise. *Journal of International Society of Sports Nutrition, 14*(20). 10.1186/s12970-017-0177-8

Khalaf, D., Krüger, M., Wehland, M., Infanger, M., & Grimm, D. (2019). The Effects of Oral l-Arginine and l-Citrulline Supplementation on Blood Pressure. *Nutrients, 11*(7), 1679. https://doi.org/10.3390/nu11071679

Kim, S. H., & Park, M. J. (2017). Effects of growth hormone on glucose metabolism and insulin resistance in human. *Annals of pediatric endocrinology & metabolism, 22*(3), 145–152. https://doi.org/10.6065/apem.2017.22.3.145

Kim, T. W., Jeong, J. H., & Hong, S. C. (2015). The impact of sleep and circadian disturbance on hormones and metabolism. *International journal of endocrinology, 2015*, 591729. https://doi.org/10.1155/2015/591729

Leproult, R., & Van Cauter, E. (2010). Role of sleep and sleep loss in hormonal release and metabolism. *Endocrine development, 17*, 11–21. https://doi.org/10.1159/000262524

Levy, E., & Chu, T. (2019). Intermittent Fasting and Its Effects on Athletic Performance: A Review. *Current sports medicine reports, 18*(7), 266–269. https://doi.org/10.1249/ JSR.0000000000000614

Mann, J., Cummings, J., Winter, N., Mete, E., & Te Morenga, L. (2022, February 26). *Carbohydrate quality and human health: a series of systematic reviews and meta-analyses*. Retrieved August 23, 2022, from https://www.thelancet.com/journals/lancet/article/PIIS0140-6736(18)31809-9/fulltext

Mathew, A. A., & Panonnummal, R. (2021). 'Magnesium'-the master cation-as a drug-possibilities and evidences. *Biometals : an international journal on the role of metal ions in biology, biochemistry, and medicine, 34*(5), 955–986. https://doi.org/10.1007/s10534-021-00328-7

Mayo Clinic. (2021). *Dietary fat: Know which to choose*. Mayo Clinic. Retrieved August 23, 2022, from https://www.mayoclinic.org/healthy-lifestyle/nutrition-and-healthy-eating/in-depth/fat/art-20045550

McClave, S. A., & Snider, H. L. (2001, March). Dissecting the energy needs of the body. Current Opinion in Clinical Nutrition and Metabolic Care. *Need Title, 4*(2), 143-147.

Mihrshahi, S., Ding, D., Gale, J., Allman-Farinelli, M., Banks, E., & Bauman, A. E. (2017). Vegetarian diet and all-cause mortality: Evidence from a large population-based Australian cohort - the 45 and Up Study. PubMed. Retrieved August 23, 2022, from https://pubmed.ncbi.nlm.nih.gov/28040519/

Morita, M., Hayashi, T., Ochiai, M., Maeda, M., Yamaguchi, T., Ina, K., & Kuzuya, M. (2014). Oral supplementation with a combination of L-citrulline and L-arginine rapidly increases plasma L-arginine concentration and enhances NO bioavailability. *Biochemical and biophysical research communications, 454*(1), 53–57. https://doi.org/10.1016/j.bbrc.2014.10.029

National Library of Medicine. (2022, June 22). *Facts about trans fats*. MedlinePlus. Retrieved August 23, 2022, from https://medlineplus.gov/ency/patientinstructions/000786.htm

Park, S. Y., Oh, M. K., Lee, B. S., Kim, H. G., Lee, W. J., Lee, J. H., Lim, J. T., & Kim, J. Y. (2015). The Effects of Alcohol on Quality of Sleep. *Korean journal of family medicine, 36*(6), 294–299. https://doi.org/10.4082/kjfm.2015.36.6.294

Pietilä, J., Helander, E., Korhonen, I., Myllymäki, T., Kujala, U. M., & Lindholm, H. (2018). Acute Effect of Alcohol Intake on Cardiovascular Autonomic Regulation During the First Hours of Sleep in a Large Real-World Sample of Finnish Employees: Observational Study. *JMIR mental health, 5*(1), e23. https://doi.org/10.2196/mental.9519

Rasch, B., & Born, J. (2013). About sleep's role in memory. *Physiological reviews, 93*(2), 681–766. https://doi.org/10.1152/physrev.00032.2012

Reinagel, M. (2016, April 8). How Trackers Can Sabotage Weight Loss. HuffPost. Retrieved August 23, 2022, from https://www.huffpost.com/entry/how-trackers-can-sabotage-weight-loss_b_9642104

Reutrakul, S., & Van Cauter, E. (2018). Sleep influences on obesity, insulin resistance, and risk of type 2 diabetes. *Metabolism: clinical and experimental, 84*, 56–66. https://doi.org/10.1016/j.metabol.2018.02.010

Sharma, S., & Kavuru, M. (2010). Sleep and metabolism: an overview. *International journal of endocrinology, 2010*, 270832. https://doi.org/10.1155/2010/270832

Suzuki, T., Morita, M., Hayashi, T., & Kamimura, A. (2017). The effects on plasma L-arginine levels of combined oral L-citrulline and

L-arginine supplementation in healthy males. *Bioscience, biotechnology, and biochemistry, 81*(2), 372–375. https://doi.org/10.1080/09168451.2016.1230007

Suzuki, I., Sakuraba, K., Horiike, T., Kishi, T., Yabe, J., Suzuki, T., Morita, M., Nishimura, A., & Suzuki, Y. (2019). A combination of oral L-citrulline and L-arginine improved 10-min full-power cycling test performance in male collegiate soccer players: a randomized crossover trial. *European journal of applied physiology, 119*(5), 1075–1084. https://doi.org/10.1007/s00421-019-04097-7

Thomas, D., Erdman, K., & Burke, L. (2016, Mar). American College of Sports Medicine Joint Position Statement. Nutrition and Athletic Performance. *Medicine & Science in Sports & Exercise, 48*(3), 543-68.

Thomas, D., KA, E., & Burke, L. (2016, Mar). Position of the Academy of Nutrition and Dietetics, Dietitians of Canada, and the American College of Sports Medicine: Nutrition and Athletic Performance. *The Journal of the Academy of Nutrition and Dietetics, 77*(1), 54. 10.3148/cjdpr-2015-047. PMID: 26917108

Van Horn, L. (2022, February 26). Fiber, Lipids, and Coronary Heart Disease A Statement for Healthcare Professionals From the Nutrition Committee, American Heart Association. ,Fiber, Lipids, and Coronary Heart Disease A Statement for Healthcare Professionals From the Nutrition Committee, American Heart Association. Retrieved August 23, 2022, from https://www.ahajournals.org/doi/10.1161/01.CIR.95.12.2701

Wynn, T. (2013, November 22). The Truth About the Caveman Diet. Psychology Today. Retrieved August 23, 2022, from https://www.psychologytoday.com/us/blog/how-think-neandertal/201311/the-truth-about-the-caveman-diet

Yin, J., Jin, X., Shan, Z., Li, S., Huang, H., Li, P., Peng, X., Peng, Z., Yu, K., Bao, W., Yang, W., Chen, X., & Liu, L. (2017). Relationship of Sleep Duration With All-Cause Mortality and Cardiovascular Events: A Systematic Review and Dose-Response Meta-Analysis of Prospective Cohort Studies. *Journal of the American Heart Association, 6*(9), e005947. https://doi.org/10.1161/JAHA.117.005947